ERECTED BY THE PHILADELPHIA CONTRIBUTORS
IN MEMORY OF THE DOCTORS, DRUGGISTS AND
NURSES OF THIS CITY WHO VOLUNTEERED
TO AID THE SUFFERERS BY THE YELLOW FEVER
AT NORFOLK & PORTSMOUTH VA. AND DIED IN THE
DISCHARGE OF THEIR DUTIES

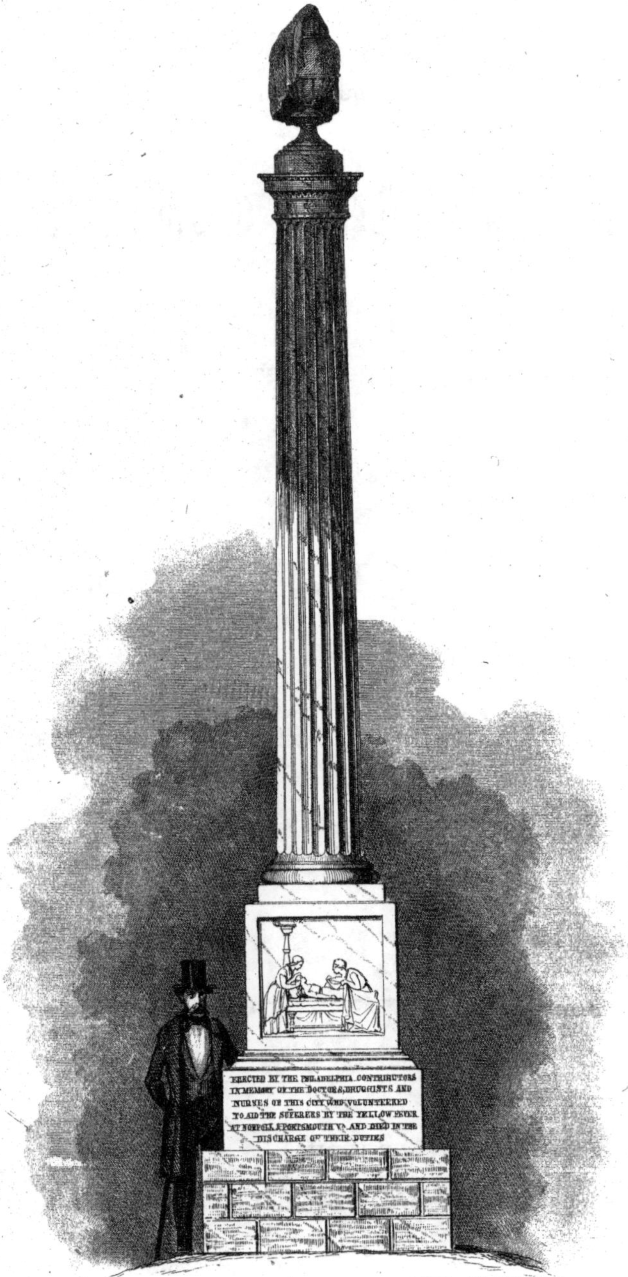

John Baird sculp. D. Chillas lith. 50 S. 3. St. Phila.

REPORT

OF THE

Philadelphia Relief Committee,

APPOINTED TO COLLECT FUNDS

FOR THE

SUFFERERS BY YELLOW FEVER,

At Norfolk & Portsmouth, Va.,

1855.

PHILADELPHIA:

INQUIRER PRINTING OFFICE, 57 SOUTH THIRD STREET

1856.

MONUMENT.

THIS memorial of the high esteem felt by the Philadelphia Contributors to the Norfolk and Portsmouth Relief Fund, for the volunteers of this city, who heroically devoted themselves to the assistance of those plague-stricken communities, and died while toiling in their labors of love, is under construction and is expected to be completed and set up in the new grounds lately opened immediately adjoining and attached to the North Laurel Hill Cemetery, by the 1st of March next.

The design, as shown by the Frontispiece, and herein described, is by JOHN BAIRD, of *Ridge Avenue*, after the suggestions of the Committee.

It is a Roman Doric Column, twenty-five feet high, including pedestal and base, and with the exception of one block, is constructed of the best Italian Marble.

The base, of Pennsylvania Marble, measures five feet and six inches square, and weighs over five tons, on which rests the pedestal base, with its richly carved moldings and appropriate inscriptions. The die or pedestal is a cube of three feet, of the best Carrara Marble, the four panels of which are enriched with elaborate carvings in *Basso Relievo*, emblematic of the Professional zeal and practical philanthropy of the entombed.

From the pedestal rises the fluted column, with its molded base and graceful capital, the whole surmounted by a shrouded Urn. The plinth of the column is inscribed. The whole work is to be carried out in the best style of art.

NORTH FRONT.

The plinth of the column bears the inscription:

As for man, his days are as grass; as a flower of the field so he flourisheth.

Psalms, CIII, 15.

The pedestal has a

CARVING

IN

BASSO RELIEVO

OF

Laying out the Dead.

The base of the Pedestal bears the inscription:

ERECTED by the Philadelphia Contributors, in memory of the Doctors, Druggists and Nurses of this City, who volunteered to aid the sufferers by Yellow Fever, at Norfolk and Portsmouth, Virginia, and died in the discharge of their duties---Martyrs in the cause of humanity.

SOUTH FRONT.

On the plinth of the column is inscribed

And let us not be weary in well-doing; for in due season we shall reap, if we faint not.

Paul to Galatians, VI, 9.

The pedestal has a

CARVING

IN

BASSO RELIEVO

OF

Hippocrates declining the Bribe.

On the base of the pedestal is inscribed:

I was sick and ye visited me.
Verily I say unto you, Inasmuch as ye have done it unto one of these least of these my brethren, ye have done it unto me.

Matthew, XXV, 36, 40.

EAST FRONT.

The plinth of the column bears the inscription:

If ye fulfil the royal law, according to the scripture, Thou shalt love thy neighbor as thyself, ye do well.

James, II. 8.

The pedestal has a

CARVING

IN

BASSO RELIEVO

OF

Charity.

On the base of the pedestal is inscribed:

THE Pestilence to which those here entombed fell martyrs, broke out at Portsmouth and Norfolk, Virginia, in July, 1855, and prevailed with great malignancy during August, September and the early part of October; attended by a mortality equal to anything hitherto observed in the United States.

WEST FRONT.

On the plinth of the column is inscribed:

Greater love hath no man than this, that a man lay down his life for his friends.

John, XV. 13.

The pedestal has a

CARVING

IN

BASSO RELIEVO

OF

The Good Samaritan.

On the Base of the pedestal are the names of the Martyrs.

Robert H. Graham, Nurse,	Aged 27
Thomas W. Handy, Druggist,	" 19
John O'Brien, Nurse,	42
E. Perry Miller, Drug. & Stu.,	" 21
A. Jackson Thompson, Nurse,	" 26
Dr. Courtlen Cole,	" 31
Mrs. Olive Whittier, Nurse,	" 55
Dr. Thomas Craycroft,	" 30
Singleton Mercer, Nurse,	Aged 35
Edmund R. Barrett, Student,	" 28
Frederick Muhsfeldt, Nurse,	" 42
Henry Spriggman, Nurse,	" 49
Dr. Herman Kierson,	" 28
Miss Lucy Johnson, Nurse,	" 25
James Hennessy, Nurse,	" 54

NOTE.

The publication of this Report and Account Current has been unavoidably delayed. Numerous requests having been made to the Committee for a correct return of the ravages of the epidemic, the authorities of Portsmouth and Norfolk were addressed on the subject, but they have not yet been able to make up a statement with the precision that is desirable. All that is known of the daily and aggregate mortality, number of cases and exact population of each place, will be found in the Appendix.

Many contributors have expressed a desire to have the correspondence of the Committee published with the report, and some of whom have sent special communications requesting it.

To publish the whole correspondence (numbering near two thousand letters and communications), is out of the question, but in order to comply with the requests preferred, a few of the letters are published along with other matter in an Appendix.

December 22, 1855.

ERRATA.

Page 81, first line, for amount brought forward, $37,586 01, read $37,756 57.
Page 81, 18th line, for balance held as a contingent fund, $391 58, read $391 48.
Page 94, 9th line, 7th word, for on, read Norfolk.
Page 111, 2d line from bottom, for copy, read reply.

REPORT.

The Committee of Relief, appointed in August last, to collect the bounty of this community, and to distribute it to the sufferers by the Yellow Fever at Portsmouth and Norfolk, Va., in submitting their account current to the public, beg leave to allude to the outbreak of the disease, and to give a short narrative of their labors:

Portsmouth and Norfolk, situate on opposite shores of the Elizabeth River, surrounded by a low, flat country, though visited by the Yellow Fever in former years, have not been recently noted for any peculiar unhealthiness. Improvement and extension, in a business point of view, have marked both places of late years. The population, including the suburb of Gosport, by the census of 1850, was twenty-two thousand, nine hundred and fifty-two; but at the breaking out of the fever, is variously estimated at from 26,000 to 29,000.

Yellow Fever had not prevailed, *epidemically*, since 1821.—On the 6th June, the steamer Ben Franklin arrived at Norfolk from St. Thomas; and, being from a suspected port, was detained at quarantine till the 19th June; after which, she was permitted to go to Gosport for repairs. No sickness occurred on her while at quarantine, and the two deaths which had taken place on board, during her voyage, are described by Dr. Fenner, of New Orleans,* as resulting from disease of the heart, in one case, and exhaustion in the other.

On the 8th July, she was ordered back to quarantine, in consequence of a case of yellow fever having occurred in Portsmouth, which the authorities thought was traceable to her.—This was the first case noticed. Dr. Schoolfield, of Portsmouth, however, on the 15th October last, personally informed the chairman of this Committee, that on the 24th June, he was

* On Yellow Fever of Norfolk and Portsmouth, Va., by E. D. Fenner, M. D., page 7.

called to visit Mrs. Fox, lately from Camden, N. J., at her residence on a farm, about a mile and a half from the town, whom he found suffering under an attack of Yellow Fever, which terminated fatally, by black vomit, on the 29th. Mrs. Fox had not been in town, or held any communication with the ship.—This case occurred nine days before the case noticed which prompted the removal of the steamer, and is not traceable to her, unless the small creek, which bordered Mrs. Fox's farm, and which emptied opposite to the Ben Franklin's anchorage, may be supposed to have borne infection on its tidal course.—Other cases followed, "particularly in a row of houses occupied by twenty-five families; these houses were very much overcrowded, and particularly filthy."

The disease continued to spread, though, "up to August 1st, there had been no case which could not be traced to Gosport. On that day it made its first appearance in Portsmouth, and spread rapidly over the town."

Norfolk, on the opposite side of the river, was not visited by the disease till the 28th July, on which day a case occurred, which has been thought to have been traced to Gosport. On the 30th July, other cases appeared in Barry's row—a locality remarkable for its insalubrity, squalidness, and the low character of its inhabitants. It is reported, however, that the late Dr. Upsher had remarked, that he had treated cases in Norfolk, early in July.

So far as your Committee can learn, there was no thorough system of sanitary measures adopted, and energetically enforced, by the harmonious action of the legislative and executive authorities of Norfolk, during the interval between the first development of the fever at Gosport, and its appearance in that city.

A strong hope that it would not cross the river, and a reliance upon the general reputation of the city for good health, appears to have imparted a feeling of security, and but few citizens removed.

The cases following those in Barry's row, either really were traced, or supposed to be, to communications with that quarter, or with Gosport and Portsmouth; and while they gave rise to further apprehension, still, there was, as yet, no general alarm. New cases, however, quickly occurred in better quarters of the city, and among the more respectable classes, and thereupon, fear and terror, amounting to panic, became dominant, impelling a general flight from the infected city.

Quarantines, with most antiquated provisions, were established by some of the adjacent counties and neighboring towns, and the affrighted people, fleeing to them for refuge, were denied a habitation. Public opinion speedily corrected this inhospitality, and regulations were adopted more in harmony with the revelations of science, and the spirit of the age.

Some of the prominent citizens who remained, organized themselves into a *Howard Association*, and heroically toiled, night and day, to mitigate the sufferings of the poor, whose humble resources had prevented escape by flight.

The fever rose rapidly, increasing in range and mortality, day after day, till its sway became almost universal, and its rates of mortality equal to anything observed in the United States. During August, it was continually on the increase in both places, and did not reach its culminating point till about the 10th September, when, after remaining stationary for several days, it, without relaxing in malignancy, slowly declined, and disappeared early in November.

D. D. FISKE, the active Mayor of Portsmouth, and the able and resolute *Sanitary Committee* of that town, HUNTER WOODIS, the energetic Mayor of Norfolk, and the *Howard Association*, presided over by the fearless WILLIAM B. FERGUSON, met the trials the havoc around imposed upon them, with unfaltering intrepidity, and unremitting industry. Their cheerful courage inspired the faint-hearted and desponding, and by their zealous activity, the aid flowing to them from all quarters of the Union, in money, medicines, and provisions, was dispensed, Hospitals organized, and the corps of devoted Doctors, Druggists, and Nurses, allotted to their duties.

All these public functionaries were stricken down with the epidemic, and two of the most prominent, HUNTER WOODIS,

Mayor, and WM. B. FERGUSON, President of the *Howard Association*, Norfolk, fell, martyrs to their over-tasked duties.

The resident Medical Corps of both towns, discharged their duties with that earnest devotion which should always be, and which happily is, predominant in the true physician. Humanity has no heroes more eminent than the profession has reared. The calm fortitude, cheerful courage, kindness, and determined energy, while living and combatting the pestilence, and patient resignation when stricken by it, of the physicians—resident and volunteer—nobly attest this.

While the press daily contained graphic accounts of the progress of the disease, and while sympathy was felt for our suffering brethren in Virginia, no appeal had been made for relief, and no authentic publication had been made, of the want and misery which was hourly arising from the suspension of the ordinary avocations of life.

Those under whose observation this distress was likely to be first manifested, felt, on the 14th August, that, though aid was still unasked, it was imperatively needed, and proceeded spontaneously to collect funds for that purpose, realizing in an hour, about six hundred dollars. In this partial movement, it was revealed on all sides, that the great heart of the community was touched, its sympathies aroused, and that nothing short of a public demonstration could satisfy the general yearning to contribute to the relief of the afflicted. Accordingly, the following call was published:—

TOWN MEETING.—A Public Meeting of the Citizens of Philadelphia will be held at the Board of Trade Room, No 30 Exchange, on THURSDAY, August 16th, at 12 o'clock precisely, to adopt measures for the Relief of the Poor of Norfolk, Portsmouth and Gosport, Virginia, now suffering under the ravages of the Yellow Fever prevailing in these towns.

MORRIS L. HALLOWELL & CO.,
BARCROFT, BEAVER & CO.,
MYERS, CLAGHORN & CO.,
S. & W. WELSH,
COPE BROTHERS,
THOMAS ALLIBONE,
G. SCULL,
THOMAS WEBSTER, JR.,
Agent Union Steamship Co.
W. M. BAIRD, and others.

In pursuance thereof, at the time appointed, the meeting organized by appointing

MORRIS L. HALLOWELL, PRESIDENT.

THOMAS ALLIBONE, WM. E. BOWEN, SAMUEL WELSH, *Vice Presidents.*

THOMAS SPARKS, JR., *Secretary.*

On motion of Thomas Webster, Jr., the following preamble and resolutions were unanimously adopted:—

Whereas, In the Providence of God, the cities of Norfolk, Portsmouth, and Gosport, Virginia, are at this time suffering under the ravages of Yellow Fever, of an epidemic and malignant type, causing a fearful mortality, and wide-spread distress; and, whereas, the citizens of said places have formed "Howard Associations" for procuring and dispensing proper aid, treatment, and attendance to the destitute; Therefore,

Resolved, That this community feels the deepest sympathy for the afflicted cities of Norfolk, Portsmouth, and Gosport, and are anxious to contribute funds to be placed at the disposal of Howard Associations, or other philanthropic bodies of those places.

Resolved, That the Chairman appoint a Committee of fifty citizens, whose duty it shall be to organize themselves into block committees, (with power to fill vacancies, or to increase their number, if necessary,) to collect funds for the relief of the aforesaid cities, and they shall appoint one of their own number as treasurer, to whom the block committee shall pay over, daily, all sums that they may collect.

Resolved, That the Chairman of the Committee, jointly with the Treasurer, shall remit, daily, if practicable, the funds reported by the Treasurer, to the "Howard Associations," or other philanthropic bodies of Norfolk, Portsmouth and Gosport, to be dispensed by them for the relief of the destitute now suffering from the pestilence, and the Chairman and Treasurer, as aforesaid, are recommended to partition each remittance according to the ratio of population of each town, as nearly as possible.

The Committee appointed under the second resolution, immediately met, increased its numbers, districted the city into blocks, and from time to time filled up vacancies, and as finally composed, of

Thomas Webster, Jr., *Chairman.*	Solomon Shepherd, *Secretary.*	Francis Grice, (*Naval Constructor.*)
Alexander J. Derbyshire	John Agnew	A. Day, (Navy Agent.)
John Trucks	Caleb Needles	J. A. Cantrell, M. D.
James C. Hand	Joseph S. Natt	John B. Austin
Jacob B. Lancaster	Hugh Craig	Wm. T. Martien
Samuel Welsh	Wharton E. Harris	George D. Parrish
Peter Thompson	Thomas J. Potts	Elliston Perot
David Faust	C. Brazer	S. Wilmer Cannell
Wm. S. Stewart	J. C. Whitall	John West
Stilwell S. Bishop	Caleb Clothier	A. B. Durand
Joseph B. Myers	A. F. Cheesebrough	J. H. Orne
Geo. H. Martin	E. Morris Buckley	Richard Vaux
Benj. B. Craycroft	J. G. Brenner	Wm. Parvin, Jr.
John D. Taylor	Solomon Bunn	J. W. Queen
Michael Dunn	M. L. Hallowell	J. W. Evans
Daniel Haddock, Jr.	Solomon Conrad	Samuel Simes
John P. Levy	Jonathan Patterson, Jr.	A. F. Glass
Hon. John Robbins	S. L. Witmer	Nathan Rowland
David Jayne, M. D.	A. Emerick	James T. Sutton
C. W. Wharton	James Graham	Jacob Naylor
Wm. A. Drown	J. B. De Haven	Wm. B. Thomas
Jay Cooke	Wm. Nassau, Jr.	John Baird
Thomas Beaver	Clayton French	M. E. Afflick
Geo. C. Presbury	Joseph Waterman	John T. Taitt
J. B. Lippincott	John Thompson	Richard George
Joseph Edwards	A. E. Outerbridge	C. J. Wistar, Jr.
Theodore Birely	S. P. Pedrick	Joseph Hansberry
Solomon Smith	J. H. Diehl	E. P. Morris
John Gibson	Wm. M. Baird	Lloyd Mifflin
Samuel Bolton	Callender I. Lewis	Edwin R. Cope
Samuel H. Bush	Samuel C. Sheppard	J. Carson
Wm. H. Inskeep	Henry C. Blair	G. W. Carpenter, Jr.
F. W. Grayson	James T. Shinn	Charles Lloyd
C. L. Sharpless	S. W. Gray	Christopher Fallon
Charles Sinickson	John Goodyear	Jesse George
Wm. E. Bowen	Arthur Howell	D. M. Fox
William Rice	George W. Brown	John Kessler, Jr.,
Charles Evans	Capt. David Teal	

steadily endeavored to collect relief for the sufferers, with what success the annexed account, in which are detailed the whole receipts and disbursements, will show.

Correspondence with the authorities of both towns was opened, and they were invited and urged to make known every want that, so far as it might lie in the power of the Committee, it should be immediately relieved. Remittances were made as rapidly as funds could be collected; and in some instances, at the outset, collections were anticipated, and remitted in advance. How gratefully they were received, the fervent letters, acknowledging the same, published in the papers of the day, have duly apprised you.

Early in September, it was evident that an incorrect impression was prevailing in the public mind, as to the true extent of the disease, and the utter inadequacy of the means of the afflicted cities to mitigate it. It was thought by many that what had been done up to that period—here and elsewhere—would be sufficient, so far as funds could be serviceable, to afford ample relief. $15,915 53 were the total collections up to that time. At a meeting of the Committee, on September 4th, on motion of J. B. Lancaster, it was

Resolved, That in view of the reported increase of the fever in Norfolk and Portsmouth, those committees who have not yet made collections, be earnestly requested to commence their duties, and prosecute them with vigor.

After various expressions of opinion, and suggestions of new modes of procuring relief, on motion of A. J. Derbyshire, it was

Resolved, That the facts revealed by the correspondence read, and telegraphic communications, be embodied in an address to the public.

In compliance with the last Resolution, the following appeal was published in all the papers of the next day:—

NORFOLK AND PORTSMOUTH SUFFERERS.

TO THE PUBLIC—A STATEMENT.—The Committee to whom the Public have confided the collection of Funds for the Relief of the Poor of Norfolk and Portsmouth, Virginia, now suffering under the ravages of Yellow Fever, find in the progress of their duty so many inaccurate impressions prevailing in the public mind, that they deem it essential to the adequate relief of those still suffering communities that a short recital should be made of facts connected with their terrible distress.

Gosport, Portsmouth and Norfolk had a population on the breaking out of this fever of about 29,000, including some hundreds of Northern mechanics working at the Navy Yard upon the two steamships of the line under construction at Gosport. In July, the propeller Ben Franklin, from St. Thomas, put into Gosport for repairs, and very shortly thereafter the mechanics working on her sickened with Yellow Fever and died. From the immediate vicinity of the dock-yard the fever spread over Gosport into adjacent Portsmouth, and, crossing the river, broke out in Norfolk—assuming a malignant and epidemic type—causing a fearful mortality—wide-spread distress and universal panic. The surrounding country and proximate towns immediately adopted the most antiquated forms of quarantine, and citizens fleeing from the pestilence were denied entrance into healthy localities, and driven back to their infected towns, even as though they had been beleaguered by a foreign foe. Public opinion has since, in some measure, corrected this inhospitality, and a less rigid quarantine has been adopted—permitting the unhappy citizens of the afflicted towns, if free from fever, to find a temporary retreat from the pestilence.

Thousands have fled, *but the Poor remain.* Flight and Death have reduced the population to less than ten thousand, and still the destroying Plague devours its *forty and fifty victims per day*—a rate of mortality truly appalling. The distress consequent upon this terrible state of affairs can hardly be described. *This, too, within sixteen hours of us*—within our power to mitigate. The gifts of TO-DAY can be made to gladden the sick and the destitute *to-morrow.* Heretofore, Philadelphia has only been called upon to relieve sister cities suffering by fever, a journey of a week or more from her limits. She has now the privilege of reaching her hand to near neighbors, and no hesitation need mark her course under the idea she will be too late. Nor should the sums sent on by Philadelphia—or the moneys received by Norfolk and Portsmouth from other sources—check the philanthrophy that ever distinguishes this community. Norfolk and Portsmouth are poor, unused to the fever. It has found them unprepared—without hospitals, bedding, medicines, or acclimated and experienced doctors and nurses. It has caused an universal panic, and suppression of the ordinary business of life. Besides sickness and death, there is poverty, and a daily dependence for food upon supplies purchased in Baltimore—*even the coffins for the dead have to be sent from* THAT CITY. Thus it will be seen that at least *five times* as much money in proportion to population *should be sent* to Norfolk and Portsmouth, as would suffice for New Orleans—where the fever is almost an annual visitation—where furnished hospitals for the purpose, an acclimated population, an experienced professional corps, and every adaptation to combat the pestilence exist. Our Virginia brethren want more aid—gratefully do they acknowledge and thank this community for its generosity, and though refraining from asking for further relief, each mail too plainly shows how much they need it.

Philanthropy is the great characteristic of Philadelphia. In some quarters she has repressed her yearning to contribute under the apprehension, it is believed, that too much might be sent. There is no such prospect existing at present. The numerous Philadelphia physicians and nurses who have volunteered their services to her sister cities, some of whom are now on the bed of sickness themselves, and others battling with the horrors of the pestilence, are children worthy of her, and should be taken care of in their perilous devotion. Hundreds of poor children have suddenly been made orphans and cry to the impoverished, despairing-plague-smitten community around them for daily sustenance. Surely there is still room for beneficence. Still work to do.

Should the liberality of this city, however, be likely to place more fund, in the treasury than the privations of our Southern brothers require, due notice will be given thereof by the Committee, and contributors will be invited to order the disposal of any such surplus as may arise.

By order of the Committee.

THOMAS WEBSTER, JR., CHAIRMAN.

SOL. SHEPHERD, SECRETARY, *pro. tem.*

Sept. 4th, 1855.

The response by the public had the effect of raising the total collections in one week to $30,028 58.

Funds continued to be actively collected, and spontaneously sent to the Committee. No relaxation was made by the Committee in their efforts to procure relief, or was any disposition evinced by the public to withhold aid so long as the fever continued its ravages. An abatement in the pestilence, and its attendant train of misery, was the signal which both the Committee and the public appeared to require to induce them to pause in their respective duties.

On October 17th, the Chairman had the pleasure of announcing that the fever was declining rapidly, and that in consequence of information received it was respectfully suggested that no further aid was needed, and that if any more funds should be contributed they would be held for the use of the orphans.

In contributing the sum of forty-six thousand dollars this community has exceeded any former effort of a similar character, and the contribution has been marked by circumstances which should not be passed by unnoticed.

No intimate or extensive business relations attached the afflicted cities to us. There was no peculiar or pecuniary tie, or any real or fancied special interests, existing between us and them. It was pure philanthropy alone, undefiled by any trace of selfishness which prompted Philadelphia to respond as she has to the sufferings of her sister cities.

While publication has been daily made of contributions from Churches, Brotherhoods, Schools and Workshops, in no instance has the name of an individual donor been published or desired to be; but numerous contributors have expressly stipulated that their names should be withheld from even the Committee.—Very many contributions have been sent in anonymously.

And so general and equal has been the charity of our citizens that the Committee have not remarked any difference in the ratio of contributions from any class. Capital has sent its liberal donation and Labor too has bestowed hers as munificently and as freely.

In reviewing the whole contribution, tracing it to the source from which it flowed, observing the cheerful alacrity with which it was given, and remembering the invitations to call for more, if more should be needed, the Committee find a pleasure which they feel will be cordially reciprocated by the public.

There has never been a fund of so large an aggregate gathered in our City for a similar purpose, nor has there ever been evinced anywhere more generous feeling for distress and spontaneous ardour to relieve it.

The capitalist, the merchant, the mechanic and the laborer; all sects, in their churches, chapels, synagogues and meeting-houses; all races, in their affiliated societies; brotherhoods of different orders in their various lodges, schools—public and private—have followed the promptings of their earnest sympathies and poured their aid into our hands. The wealthy from the country retreats have sent checks for handsome amounts, workmen in their shops and women in factories have devoted a day's earnings, and children have given their whole savings. The benevolence of our community has welled out as freely and as purely as the gushing springs of nature, and almost as inexhaustibly.

Nor was relief confined to such material aid merely as money could procure. It is with pride that Philadelphia can point to relief a hundred times more efficient which she rendered to the afflicted cities in the heroic corps of doctors, druggists and nurses, who volunteered to visit the sick and went on their errand of mercy. Sixty persons repaired to the scene of suffering, nearly all of whom were, sooner or later, attacked with the fever, and fourteen died—martyrs in the cause of humanity.

At the breaking out of the epedimic there were in Portsmouth ten practising physicians, and twenty-one in Norfolk. The duties devolving upon them exceeded the ability of twice or thrice their number to perform, and they fell before the destroyer, easy victims, in consequence of the exhaustion resulting from their overtasked duties. The first cry of distress heard here was an appeal for medical aid, and it was the first which was responded to. Dr. WM. H. FREEMAN volunteered on the 16th of August, left by the first train, and reached Norfolk on the 18th—the first volunteer physician who had set out from home and arrived there—preceded only by Dr. Stone of New Orleans, whose presence in the North had opportunely enabled him to reach Norfolk on the 17th. Other volunteers followed daily. On the 23d of August, Dr. MARTIN RIZER, with letters from this Committee, arrived at Portsmouth, being the first volunteer physician who reached that town. Aid of this important character continued to offer and to be dispatched from this city. Similar assistance was daily being received by the stricken cities from New Orleans, Mobile, Augusta, Savannah and Charleston; this, and the unwillingness of the authorities to devote to the perils of the pestilence unacclimated men and women, as they feared, whose noble impulses were impelling them from this city to their assistance, induced the Howard Association of Norfolk to decline, on September 9th, any further aid from the North, and in a few days thereafter the Sanitary Committee of Portsmouth came to a like determination.

Generous tenders of professional services from doctors, druggists and nurses, to the number of nearly one hundred, continued to be made, which the Committee reluctantly had to decline.

While the motives which actuated the authorities in refusing further professional aid from the North are in the highest degree commendable to their sense of humanity, the Committee regretted their determination, and were of the opinion that the volunteers from this city who had been seized with the fever and died, had been made the more liable to attack from the fatigues and exhaustion following their overtasked powers of endurance, and at the same time necessarily less able to withstand its ravages and recover therefrom. The Committee thought that, if permitted, they could have sent on a sufficient number to have reinforced their delegation, enabling them to partition their duties, thus making them lighter for each, and offering to all opportunities of recess for recreation and recuperation. The Committee *knew* the generosity of this community would have furnished them with the means to have maintained a numerous corps of volunteers, and finally they knew that going from this city did not necessarily make them unacclimated, as the persons whose generous offers had to be declined *had* had yellow fever during the war in Mexico, lately in South America, in the West Indies, New Orleans, and other places. The Committee believed, in short, that in a community like this, of over 500,000 souls, they could readily gather any reasonable force of resolute, skilful, acclimated professional men and women, who had had yellow fever, treated it and nursed in it.

The volunteers to Norfolk were:—

Dr. Wm. H. Freeman.
Louis Martin Y de Castro, Medical Student.
W. W. Maule, Nurse.
Captain Nathan Thompson, Nurse.
Thomas Craycroft, Medical Student.
Mrs. Ann McCaust.
Dr. James McFadden.
Dr. A. A. Zeigenfusse.
Mrs. Catherine Heck, Nurse.
Dr. Eli T. Worl.
Joseph Robertson, Nurse.
Wm. L. Driver, Nurse.
Mrs. Mary Jacoks, Nurse.
A. Judson Gibbs, Druggist.
Dr. Herman Keirson.
Thos. W. Handy, Druggist.
Lewis Kunitz, Cupper and Bleeder.
Dr. J. E. Marsh.
John O'Brien, Nurse.
Mrs. Alida Seyferell.
Henry L. Van Clieve, Druggist.
John W. Grimes, Nurse.
Thomas Whittin, Nurse.
Vincent Torres, Nurse.
Dr. A. B. Campbell.
Dr. J. R. McCoy.
Midshipman J. R. Roche, U. S. Navy, Nurse.
Andrew Jackson Johnson.

To Portsmouth.

Dr. Martin Rizer.
Thomas D. Beard, Nurse.
R. W. Graham, Nurse.
Henry Spriggman, Nurse.
James A. Boon, Nurse.
Mrs. Caroline C. Barnett, Nurse.
Dr. Courtland Cole.
Dr. J. M. C. Randel.
Dr. Geo. L. Hamill.
Dr. J. D. Bryant.
Singleton Mercer, Nurse.
Mrs. Margaret Kinnin, Nurse.
John Flood, Nurse.
Edwin R. Barrett, Medical Student.
Frederick Mushfeldt, Cupper and Bleeder.
Dr. T. F. Azpell.
E. Perry Miller, Druggist.
Charles D. Shreive, Druggist.
Dr. Ralph L. Briggs.
Theodore C. Stryker, Nurse.
John Wells, "
Mrs. Olivee Whittier, "
Miss Leonora Patterson, "
Dr. Stewart Kennedy.
Capt. James Johnson, Nurse.
James Hennesy, "
William Hersen, "
S. E. Townsend, "
James E. Gordon, Druggist.
D. J. W. Molle.
Alexander Ytasse, Nurse.
William Parker, "

The names of those who died are:—

Thomas Craycroft, Medical Student.
Robert W. Graham, Nurse.
Henry Spriggman, "
Thomas W. Handy, Druggist.
E. Perry Miller, "
Singleton Mercer, Nurse.
Dr. Herman Keirson.
Edwin R. Barrett, Student.
Mrs. Olive Whittier, Nurse.
William Herson "
Dr. Courtland Cole.
Frederick Murfeldt, Cupper and Bleeder.
John O'Brien, Nurse.
Miss Lucy Johnson,* Nurse.
Andrew Jackson Johnson, Nurse.

The highest commendations have been passed by the authorities of Portsmouth and Norfolk, upon the skill, humanity and courage of the delegation from this city.

All the resident physicians of Portsmouth and Norfolk, thirty-one in number, had the fever, and *fourteen* died. In Portsmouth "twenty-six of the thirty-two physicians, resident and volunteers, had the fever, and ten of the twenty-six died—a mortality of thirty-eight per cent." The ratio of the number attacked, of resident and volunteer physicians in Norfolk, to their whole number, and the ratio of mortality are not known, but it is believed to be rather less than at Portsmouth; nor have the Committee sufficient data to compute the ratio of mortality among the druggists and nurses of either place, but it is believed to exceed the ratio in the number attacked as well as in the mortality observed among the physicians.

If doctors, druggists and nurses are to be ranked as the commissioned officers to combat pestilence, a comparison will

* This young lady was advised to remain home, and her application declined on the ground of her apparently feeble constitution.

show that the mortality in their ranks in the Portsmouth and Norfolk campaign exceeds the mortality among the regular officers of the Russian and Allied armies in the campaigns of the Crimea. If there was heroic courage shown in storming or defending the Malakoff, and in the attempt on the Redan, it required yet more to minister to the sick and dying in the plague-stricken cities of Norfolk and Portsmouth.

The Volunteer delegation offered their aid from the highest motives which can animate human conduct, and toiled and sickened, and some died, without the thought of fee or reward. Services such as theirs, prompted by such motives, are appreciated wherever civilization is known, but the money is not coined that could be offered in compensation for their perils, labor and love.

To afford some evidence however of the high regard in which their devotion is held by the community, the Committee resolved on October 8th, that the Chairman and Secretary should, according to their judgment and discretion, purchase suitable testimonials for each of the delegation, or place the funds at the disposal of each for that purpose. Accordingly, in pursuance of this resolution, the sum of thirty-five hundred dollars has been charged for the purpose aforesaid, and has either been handed over to the members of the delegation or is held in trust to pay for silver plate and other testimonials for such as gave their preference to that form of the evidence of the esteem of their fellow-citizens.

To the widows of the deceased there has been presented the sum of one hundred and eighty dollars, and the further sum of four hundred dollars is held in trust for them, which sum will be somewhat augmented by the gift of one of the physicians, who has declined any other testimonial than a letter of thanks, and has relinquished the value of the gift proffered to him to the widows and orphans of the deceased Philadelphia volunteers.

The families of the deceased volunteers are anxious to have their remains brought home. They can be identified, and the

Committee have promised to have it done in the coming mid-winter. The Union Steamship Company will bring them on without charge, and the Laurel Hill Cemetery Company have kindly offered a suitable lot for their re-interment. The Committee have placed the sum of two thousand dollars in the hands of its chairman, as trustee, to defray the unavoidable expenses attending the removal and re-interment of the bodies, and to erect a suitable marble monument over them commemorative of their devoted heroism.

The trustee waits only for the adoption of this recommenda tion to make the necessary arrangements to fulfil the promises made to their relatives.

It may be but proper here to state, that testimonials for their noble services, if computed by the same rules which governed the distribution to the living, would require a sum not much less than has been put in trust for the vault, expenses of burial and monument. They have fallen in the cause of humanity—no sacrifice so noble. In the words of the evangelist, "Greater love hath no man than this, that he lay down his life for his friends."

Theirs was a common fate. Let then one tomb contain their hallowed remains, and one testimonial commemorate their virtues and attest our remembrance of them. The living are honored, we should not allow the dead to be forgotten.*

The account hereunto annexed shows that there has been remitted to Norfolk in cash $14,503 33

And to Portsmouth 10,302 21

The Committee, in view of the almost total cessation of business, and the general want of supplies of merchandise at Norfolk and Portsmouth, and with the full knowledge that for the greater part of their daily food the desolated cities were dependent upon supplies purchased in Baltimore and Richmond, and

* Upon the adoption of the Report of the committee by the public meeting, the chairman contracted with John Baird of Ridge Avenue for this structure, and it is now being cut and constructed and will be completed about the first of March next. A full description of its style and character will be found in the Appendix. The Lithographic print of it—from the original design —which forms the frontispiece of this pamphlet, was generously presented by David Chillas Esq., Lithographer, No. 47 South Third street.

forwarded to them by the steamboats plying in the Chesapeake and the James Rivers, invited the authorities to communicate their wants to them, in order that they might be relieved at once. Without waiting for orders, the Committee bought and sent on various medicines, articles of diet and alleviatives for the sick; and were pleased to find, in many instances, they had been able to anticipate the wishes of the authorities. This, too, was fortunately the case with regard to druggists and apothecaries —three having been sent on with letters of introduction, and arrived there the same day that the need of assistance in the dispensaries was first felt.

With a view of executing the orders sent on to the Committee promptly, and to be assured of care in the transit and delivery, the proffer of the services of Captain Nathan Thompson, a convalescent volunteer nurse, was accepted, and he was made the steward and travelling agent of the Committee.

A large part of the invoices of merchandise which were sent on to both places, as per account annexed, was bought under his supervision, and forwarded under his charge. In every instance the purchases were made for cash, and in very many cases no advance over cost was asked by the sellers, and further liberal concessions were made for the benefit of the fund upon settlement being made. By the kindness of the Philadelphia, Wilmington and Baltimore Rail Road Company, not only were volunteers passed over their road free, but at considerable inconvenience, as well as expense to the Company, room was furnished, without charge, on the express mail train at 1 o'clock, P.M. daily, for the stores of merchandise bought for the sufferers, thus enabling the Committee to connect with the boats of the Baltimore Steam Packet Company, and place the means of relief in Norfolk in sixteen hours. Too much praise cannot be bestowed upon the liberality of these two corporations.

The Committee, in view of the universal interest which has been manifested in this city in the late calamitous visitation, resolved that a clear, full, and detailed Report and Account Current should be submitted to the public, and, unwilling to further tax the generosity of the press, and at the same time believing that the subject was worthy of publication in a form which might be preserved, have ordered five thousand copies of this Report and annexed Account to be printed in pamphlet form and distributed among the contributors to the fund.

Whatever sum may remain after the trusts for building the monument for the dead and purchasing testimonials for the living shall have been fulfilled, will, with whatever surplus there may arise from the contingent fund and all further contributions, be invested in Philadelphia six per cent loan for the benefit of the orphans.

At the *request* of the chairman, on motion of A. J. Derbyshire, an auditing committee was appointed, on October 24th, to examine and audit the chairman's account.

The following is their report:—

"We the undersigned, a committee appointed to audit the account of Thomas Webster, Jr., Chairman of the Committee of Relief for the Norfolk and Portsmouth Sufferers, report that we have examined his accounts, and find that he has received the sum of forty-five thousand eight hundred and fourteen dollars and forty-six cents, and that he has disbursed thirty-seven thousand seven hundred and eleven dollars and fifty-three cents, leaving a balance on hand of eight thousand one hundred and two dollars and eighty-nine cents, of which balance the sum of eight thousand and thirty-four dollars and twenty cents is in the Farmers' and Mechanics' Bank, and the remainder in change.*

ALEX. J. DERBYSHIRE,
J. B. LANCASTER,
THOS. SPARKS, JR.

Philada. Nov. 21, 1855.

Reference to the amount will show that a fund of Three Thousand dollars has been ordered to be invested in Philadelphia six per cent loan, to be remitted to the contemplated Orphans' Asylum of Norfolk and Portsmouth, as soon as they shall be incorporated, and their managers elected.†

* Sixty-eight dollars and fifty-nine cents has been received since 21st November and added to the above.

† The Chairman has made the investment, and holds the Certificates of loan in trust, for the purpose aforesaid.

It is with pride that the Committee point to the gratifying fact that our own children have taken the initiative in this matter, not only as among the Philadelphia contributors, but as regards the whole Union. It is believed they were the first to collect and send in funds to be set apart for the permanent benefit of the Orphans. Charity in this case, like the quality of mercy,

> "Is twice blessed;
> It blesseth him that gives, and him that takes."

The unprompted benevolence of our children at School—particularly in the Public Schools—reflects the highest merit on them, their preceptors and parents, evincing as it does, that the culture of the affections, and the education of the heart, have been as carefully regarded as the development and training of the mind is known to be. The industry of the girls in getting up garments for the orphans, and other sufferers, and the devotion of their savings, along with the boys' subscriptions, show how well they have learned one of the great lessons of life—to feel for the sufferings of humanity, and to relieve them.

Contributions from some of the Protestant Episcopal, the Catholic, and other churches, from individuals, from the Employees of the Columbia Railroad, Employees of the Philadelphia, Wilmington, and Baltimore Railroad, from Odd Fellows, and various other sources, in cash, and contributions in clothing, in medicines, provisions, &c., to a considerable extent, estimated to be equal to $6000, were despatched by the donors, direct, without the agency of this Committee.

If this were added to the total contributions, and the amounts received from New Jersey and other States *deducted* therefrom, the aggregate of the Philadelphia contribution would be over . .	$50,000
And add thereto the contribution of Pittsburg, ...	2,792
" " " Lancaster, ...	2,103
York, Harrisburg, Columbia, Easton, and various other parts of the State, sent direct, or through the Baltimore Committee, estimated to be at least	10,000
Would show the total contribution of Pennsylvania to be about .	65,000

The Committee do not refer to the liberality of our city and State with any boastful or vain-glorious feeling, but with honest pride, and point in the spirit of congratulation to the many proofs afforded, that both city and State maintain their well-established reputation for philanthropy, and preserve undiminished the pure and true character, stamped upon them by their great founder, for Brotherly Love.

Indeed, there is yet a wider field of rejoicing, and without limits—geographical or political—to congratulations; for not we alone, but all cities and all States of the Union responded to the cry of affliction. The wail of woe which went forth from the seaboard cities of Virginia thrilled throughout the land, and the whole Union beat with responsive sympathy—proving us to be a people, one in feeling, and one in patriotism.

Our report as a Committee of Relief here ends.

One duty yet remains. Pestilential Yellow Fever, a subject of melancholy importance in the annals of Philadelphia, raging with almost unparalleled malignancy during the past summer and autumn, within three hundred miles of us, naturally recalls to mind the history of our desolations in 1793 and 1798, and prompts the consideration of our exposure to the fresh assaults of the destroyer.

Vague and indefinite apprehensions have been remarked among us, and the idea that the disease is migrating northwardly, has been published and adopted by some. Dr. Nott, of Mobile, in 1853—in his communication upon the epidemic of that year, addressed to the Sanitary Commission of New Orleans—remarks: "I shall be greatly deceived if the same disease does not attack cities on the Atlantic next season—*and particularly Philadelphia.*"*

And further, in support of this theory of the *transportability* of the disease and its migratory character, after narrating several facts, he observes, "this fact, and others, lead me strongly to believe that Philadelphia will be scourged next summer, and probably other Atlantic Cities."† Fortunately, he has

* Report of Sanitary Commission on Yellow Fever of 1853, published by authority of Common Council of New Orleans, page 96.
† Ibid, page 102.

been "greatly deceived." The same writer, in a letter dated 19th August last, published in the Charleston Mercury, remarking on the fever then desolating Norfolk and Portsmouth, re-affirms his convictions. Publication in the newspapers of this and similar predictions of the migratory character of the disease, and our *pre-disposition* to attack, have given a wide prevalence to the idea that we may look for the visitation of this pestilence next season; and, therefore, the question of our pre-disposition, or the lesser one of our liability to attack by Yellow Fever, should not be idly dismissed.

That this dreadful disease has prevailed here in epidemic form, attended by frightful devastation, time and again, is a matter of history. It has re-appeared after an interval of as long as *thirty-three years*, and has been as malignant here as in any other part of the United States.

Of the disease itself, but very little more is known of its true therapeutical treatment now than in the last century. Dr. Stone, of New Orleans, a writer of authority and a practitioner of great skill and experience in the disease, in a recent discourse before the New York Academy of Medicine, says:—

"Yellow Fever is a self-limited disease; it is not to be treated; it is to be managed." The latest experience shows it still baffles the art of the faculty, and, defying all remedial agents, carrys off 33 to 75 per cent. of all whom it attacks. While so little has been learned of its proper treatment, there has happily been some progress made in the true knowledge of its causation, and consequently of the means and appliances of *preventing* its development.

That it *originated* here in 1699, 1741, 1747, 1762, 1793, 1794, 1797, 1798, 1799, 1802, 1803, 1805, 1820, and in 1853, from natural causes existing in our midst, and was not *imported* by any vessel from the tropics, the larger number of the faculty do not *now* doubt. The last visitation, in 1853, happily but a slight one as regards the number attacked, but malignant in itself, as marked by a mortality of 75 per cent., though ascribed at the time by many, and even now by some, to importation by the Barque Mandarin, from Cienfuegos, Cuba, is by the latest writer on Yellow Fever, and the highest known authority—La Roche—directly charged to the non-observance of proper sanitary conditions. Dr. Wilson Jewell, the eminent President of the Board of Health, who was the chronicler of this epidemic, and disposed to attribute it to the Barque, says: "The docks along the Delaware line, between Lombard and Almond Streets, as usual, contained large accumulations of mud and other filth." Again, he says, "In addition to the prevalence of the morbific atmosphere on board the Mandarin, we must not for a moment conceal the existing causes in the immediate vicinity of South Street Wharf, sufficient to justify the supposition of their agency in the development of disease of a malignant type, when subjected to the high thermometrical influence which prevailed throughout the months of June and July. Not the least mischievous of these causes in the production of an unhealthy atmosphere, was the outlet of a sewer into the dock at South Street Ferry—belching forth continually putrid masses of animal and vegetable filth accumulating around its mouth, and exposed at low water to the rays of a burning sun, exhaling streams of poisonous gases into the surrounding air." And again he says: "The whole neighborhood, however, may be considered as favorable to the production and nourishment of malarious fevers, in view of its proximity to the river docks, the open sewer at South Street Wharf, the damp cellars, filthy alleys, and other local causes of disease, under such a long-continued high thermometrical atmosphere as prevailed in the months of July, August and September."*

The local origin of the epidemic of this year may be considered a settled point, disputed by but few of the faculty, or reasoning inquirers after its true history. In a paper by Dr. La Roche, read to the College of Physicians of Philadelphia, April 5th, 1854, there is a clear statement of a well marked case of Yellow Fever, made from the note-book of Dr. Keating, the attendant physician, which terminated fatally on the 6th

* Yellow Fever. By La Roche, Vol. 2d, page 795.

of July, *seven days before the arrival of the Mandarin* at the wharf, and thirteen days before the first suspicious case was observed in the neighborhood of South Street Wharf,* which it is difficult to account for on any other hypothesis than that of local origin.

The dreadful epidemics of 1793, 1798, 1799, were, as usual, attributed to importation; and during that of 1793, a general belief of its contagiousness prevailed. Dr. Rush, and other eminent men of that period, upon patient investigation and comparison, renounced the idea of contagion, attacked it, and overthrew the horrible phantom, under whose abominable rule parents and children, husband and wife, so often forgot their instincts and their duties. And going further, Rush, Caldwell and others, charged the existence of the fever "to putrid exhalations arising from decomposed animal and vegetable substances;" to the filthy state of Pegg's Run, Dock Creek, and the neighborhood of the Drawbridge, and various other morbific influences arising from the numerous imperfections in the drainage of the streets, their unpaved condition, filthy state of the docks, numerous ponds of stagnant water adjacent to the city, and lastly, to the "want of a good supply of pure water."

Under the admonition of such terrible visitations as 1793, 1798, and 1799, improvement in the Hygienic condition of the city proceeded with spirit. Streets were paved, Dock Creek arched over, and water introduced. To these reforms may, in some degree, be attributed the restrained spread of the disease, and its diminished mortality in 1802, 1803, and 1805.—Notwithstanding the increased improvements in hygienic conditions in a general way, the fever became again epidemic in 1819 and 1820. In its visitation in the latter year, it broke out in Water Street, and in a range of frame buildings on the north side of Hodge's Dock and Wharf, in the vicinity of Race Street. "This dock," says Dr. Jackson's account,† "has been neglected for some years, and at low water (it is at present) uncovered nearly its whole extent, and a large mass of mud, of animal and vegetable remains are thus exposed to the action

* Transactions of College of Philadelphia Physicians, page 247, Vol.
† Account of the Yellow Fever in 1820, by Samuel Jackson, M. D., page 16.

of the sun and air. Two tunnels, into which empty the privies of a range of buildings, discharge their contents into the dock. In the month of May, a quantity of potatoes were landed on the wharf, north of the dock, which were in a damaged state, and were extremely offensive. They were stored in the neighborhood, where they were picked, and the worst of them thrown into the river a few feet above the dock, into which a large portion were carried by the current, to add to the mass of decaying and putrescent matter already deposited there."

In the vicinity of Walnut Street Wharf, where the disease was subsequently the most prevalent, it was attributed, says the same writer, to "a quantity of damaged vegetables which were stored below Walnut Street Wharf, especially beans and potatoes. In consequence of the failure of the potato crop, the importation of that vegetable had been unusually great, such quantities, it is believed, never were before brought to this port. A very considerable part of what was imported, were on their arrival, in a very bad state, and some cargoes completely damaged. The greater part were landed and stored at Walnut Street Wharf."

Again, "in the month of June there were stored in one store in that vicinity, twenty-five hundred bushels in a damaged state. They became so disagreeable to the neighbors that they were removed in the course of that month. The store was washed out, but the *offensive smell still continued*."* "Putrefactive fermentation, arising from the dirty and foul condition of the wharves in this vicinity,"† is also strongly alluded to by the same writer; and in reference to the development in Duke Street, (then Artillery Lane,) Northern Liberties, he alludes to its proximity to what was called in a petition of that time, "the greatest nuisance in Philadelphia," Pegg's Run, and describes it "as an open culvert or common sewer, passing through the closely built parts of Penn Township, Spring Garden, and the Northern Liberties, to the River Delaware. In its course, it receives the contents of the gutters of the numerous populous streets and alleys it crosses, and two culverts

* Jackson, page 39. † Jackson, page 41.

from the city also open into it. Along its borders are situated a number of manufactories of glue, starch, dressed skins, and soap. About fifty slaughter-houses, and the privies of most of the adjoining dwellings, the refuse, fermentable and putrescent matters of which are all emptied into its stream. Except during the heavy rains, or immediately after them, the stream is barely sufficient to carry along, with a sluggish current, the mass of decomposing, offensive substances that compose it, for in fact, it seems more like liquid mud than water."* In the epidemic of 1820, the origin of which is so pointedly given by the author just quoted, "the disease differed in nothing from that of preceding times, and the mortality, in proportion to the whole number affected, was nearly as great as had been observed in the most fatal seasons."†

The returns made by the Board of Health, showed the number of cases to be one hundred and twenty-five, of which eighty-three died, a mortality of near 67 per cent. The measures adopted to arrest the spread of the disease, were attended by the happiest results. Then it was that past experience in the disease, and the recommendations of Rush and others of a preceding period were for the first time speedily and thoroughly carried out. Under the skilful energy of the efficient President of the Board of Health, Dr. Samuel Jackson, the most vigorous measures were promptly enforced, and the baleful spread of the epidemic cut short in every locality wherein it developed itself.

The Board of Health removed not only the sick to Hospitals, but resolved to clear the infected district of *all* its inhabitants. "When that measure was accomplished, fences were erected, cutting off the approach to Hodge's Wharf and Dock, which appeared to be the focus of the disease."‡

A similar plan was forthwith executed upon the first manifestation of the disease in the other localities, and had the desired effect to put a complete stop to the disease in those vicinities.

"The appearance of the Yellow Fever in a formidable form

* Jackson, page 47. † La Roche, Vol. 1, p. 106. ‡ Jackson, page 19.

after so long an interval, awakened once more the dormant apprehensions of the public generally, as well as of the Board of Health, and of the city authorities, for the future safety of the city. Public meetings were held, at which the subject was discussed, and appropriate measures suggested. By private individuals, schemes of improvement, some of great magnitude, and amounting even to the removal of all the buildings situate between the west side of Front Street to the Delaware from Vine to Fourth Streets were proposed." A joint Committee of Councils considered the subject of the late visitation, and in an elaborate report, "fully sensible of the absolute necessity of introducing some modification in the ordinances relative to the cleanliness of the city, in order to insure the existence of a pure atmosphere, which, they were aware, was no less desirable as a means of preventing the spread of malignant fevers, than as a certain alleviation of them, thought it necessary to recommend the adoption of a few of the most important schemes required for that purpose;" they suggested among other measures—

That no wharf be hereafter built, unless the dock on either side be so deep as to be covered by water at *low* tide.

That docks now made, and which are not covered at low tide, be filled up or dug deeper, to produce that effect at the head of the dock."

That Yellow Fever has originated here, is thus well attested; and that it may re-appear, should we neglect to enforce a judicious sanitary code, and by tolerating hygienic abuses invite it, is the inevitable corollary.

By well authenticated official records, and by the writings of Rush, Deveze, Caldwell, Carey, and a host of others on the epidemics of 1793–7–8; by Jackson on the Fever of 1820; La Roche on that of 1853; its development is charged to local origin, and traced to the neglect of proper observances of judicious precautions to prevent the formation and accumulation of filth, animal and vegetable, which, under the action of great and prolonged solar heat, and other predisposing influ-

*La Roche, Vol 1, p. 109.

ences, is ONE, at least, of the indisputable causes of Yellow Fever.

Are we any more circumspect and vigilant now, in 1855, with the monition of the awful ravages during the past summer within three hundred miles of us, than we were in 1820 and in 1853?

Have we now no nuisance to abate? no pest holes to obliterate? Are there not *now* docks as foul, whose putrid bottoms are as much exposed at half or low tide as was "Hodge's" in 1820? Gutters as reeking, houses as filthy, crowded, and abominable—privies as vile as those described? Are there not other runs and creeks traversing the inhabited parts of our city, as loathsome, impure and poisonous as was "Pegg's Run" in 1820? Have we not *now* other sewers, whose outlets are "belching forth continually putrid masses of animal matter," like the sewer of South Street Ferry in 1853?

With the immense increase in the population of the city, and the great expansion of its area, like all other cities, there is to be remarked a concentration, in some localities, of population attended by every privation of comfort and salubrity. Overcrowded courts, lanes, and alleys, are undoubtedly more numerous now than at any other time in our city's history. And if we possess the advantages of better drainage, paved streets and wharves, and a bountiful supply of pure water, all which our fathers of '93 and '98 were deprived of, and to whose urgent advice we may mainly attribute our possession of them, still, we have a population ten times as great, with destitution, nuisances and vices peculiar to congregated masses, and our city, improved as it is in so many respects, is necessarily, owing to its density, surrounded with an atmosphere less invigorating than when but 40,000 to 60,000 souls were its denizens.

Well may we shrink from contemplating the possible extent of the ravages of a pestilence among us, a city of half a million, at any time hereafter as malignant as that of 1793 or 1798, or that which just died out at Norfolk and Portsmouth.

The delusive doctrine of importation, it is to be remarked,

has been attended by pernicious results, inducing almost every community wherever Yellow Fever has broke out, to shut their senses to the morbific agencies existing around them, and to charge some vessel from a suspected port with introducing it, and often no power of reason, or force of demonstration, has been sufficient to correct the impression so readily and so fatally adopted. Dr. Caldwell, in speaking of the Health Authorities of 1805, says: "Such was their fanaticism on the subject of the introduction of disease from abroad, that they would at any time leave the carcass of an animal putrefying in the street, and filling the air with a poison truly pestilential, to go in search of a sailor sick only of a last night's frolic, or to meet at the Health Office for the purpose of passing a resolution to prevent the most clean and healthy West India vessel from entering our port."*

The views of those who refuse to attribute the development of Yellow Fever to such local causes as poisonous exhalation, arising from putrid decomposition and similar miasma, and who yet readily ascribe to them the secondary part of spreading it when once imported, are thus happily summed up by La Roche:*

"It is affirmed or suggested that the poison (whether introduced into a vessel during its stay in a sickly port, or elaborated in the hold or other parts matters not) when brought to a heretofore healthy place, contaminates the atmosphere of the latter, and spreads epidemically, notwithstanding the departure of that vessel, in consequence of having multiplied itself by assimilating to its own nature something it meets with there. In other words, the peculiar poisonous effluvium which, if imported into a perfectly clean locality, would occasion no evil effect, acts very differently when brought, during hot weather, to a place replete with the materials from which issue morbid effluvia; for it then plays on those materials the part of a ferment, and through their agency is enabled to reproduce itself, or out of them to give origin to a substance of the same nature, or endowed with identical properties, as yeast is generated during the vinous fermentation which yeast has set in motion."

* An Essay on Pestilential or Yellow Fever, &c. C. Caldwell, p. 42.
† Transactions of College of Philadelphia Physicians, p. 255.

It is not for this Committee to pronounce on theories of Yellow Fever, nor are they competent to do more than to allude to them. Dr. Nott's opinion of the transportability and migratory character of this fever, and his predictions regarding its future development here and at New York—the doctrine of the importationists—with or without the adjunctive fermentative theory—and the opposite teachings and opinions of the more numerous part of the faculty, who find its origin in local causes, are differences of theory for the profession to elucidate, reconcile and determine.

It is in our power, however, in taking a general view of the subject, to affirm most absolutely that there is a hearty and unanimous concurrence of testimony as to the fact that exhalations and poisonous gasses arising from vegetable and anima decomposition, *are* the morbific agents by which the fever spreads itself, and which enter into and contributes to make its type more or less malignant, and its duration less or greater, according to the degree of infectious effluvia which may exist.

Adopting, then, the language of the Report of Councils in 1821 regarding the purity of the atmosphere, "No less desirable as the means of preventing the spread of malignant fevers than as a certain alleviation of them." Let us ask if we have done all that science teaches us can be done to avert the development of this dreadful disease at any time hereafter. Let us inquire what is the hygienic condition of our city, and whether our sanitary laws are as well digested, as comprehensive, and as exact as they should be. Let each citizen in his own way calmly and closely observe for himself what nuisance or what violations of good sanitary regulations exist, and join with his neighbor in a private or public movement to correct whatever abuses may be detected and relax no effort until reform is enforced and the nuisances abated. The authorities of the city are vigilant, and will be the more so if their constitnents are observing, active and determined. The Board of Health are ever ready to notice communications made to them of abuses, and invoke the scrutiny and co-operation of citizens in maintaining the wholesome condition of the city.

There may be, and indeed there is, strong ground to believe that there are nuisances now existing, such as foul docks, and mouths of sewers exposed at low tide, open and unarched creeks and runs—foul and fetid—which demand immediate attention, the reform and improvement of which should be commenced forthwith under a low stage of solar heat while there is the least liability of an injurious effect resulting from disturbing masses of filth.

Improvements in our hygienic condition it is thought, too, would follow the enactment of good laws forbidding the storage of certain vegetable matter during the summer months, and in establishing public slaughter-houses, or *abbattiors*. It is not for this Committee to suggest any plan of reform, they feel that their duty will be discharged in pointedly calling attention to the subject of sanitary regulations as a means of averting pestilential yellow fever and other malarious diseases hereafter among us.

One of the best evidences of the highest civilization is revealed in the sanitary laws of a people—are we prepared for this test? Philadelphia has, indeed, led the van in sanitary reforms in the United States, owing possibly to her great devastations of '93 and '98. She claims to be, and justly is, the seat and fountain head of Medical Science; and has thus her reputation and her pride to prompt, and in the calamities of Norfolk and Portsmouth fresh monitions to hasten her forward in devising and enforcing a perfect code of sanitary laws. The British Parliament have been and are elaborating in their "Health of Towns Bill," a system of hygienic reforms—the rapid concentration of population in masses is one of the features of the age and demands it. Let us then, for our comfort and prosperity—for our health and our lives—look around, investigate, consult and combine to avert a pestilential epidemic at any time hereafter by whatever may now be done by human agency.

THOMAS WEBSTER, Jr. *Chairman.*

A Public Meeting of the Philadelphia Contributors to the Norfolk and Portsmouth Fund was held on the evening of the 29th November, in pursuance of a call of the Committee of Relief, at the Assembly Buildings. M. L. HALLOWELL Presided, and *Thomas Sparks, Jr.* and *Wharton E. Harris* acted as Secretaries. A lengthy Report and an elaborate Account Current were submitted from the Committee, through their Chairman, MR. WEBSTER, which was, on motion, unanimously accepted and the Committee discharged.

Mr. Alexander J. Derbyshire offered the following resolution:

Resolved, That the self-sacrificing devotion and marked administrative ability displayed by THOMAS WEBSTER, JR. Esq., Chairman of the Relief Committee, in the discharge of his arduous and delicate duties, merit the highest praise of this community—which was unanimously adopted.

Mr. Jacob B. Lancaster offered the following resolution:—

Resolved, That the thanks of this meeting be returned to the editors of the different newspapers of the city for their liberality in publishing all communications and advertisements of the Committee free of charge—which was unanimously adopted.

On motion of Mr. D. S. Winebrenner, the proceedings of this meeting were ordered to be printed along with the Report and Account Current of the Committee.

MORRIS L. HALLOWELL, *President.*

THOMAS SPARKS JR.,
WHARTON E. HARRIS, } *Secretaries.*

ACCOUNT CURRENT

OF THE

CHAIRMAN OF THE RELIEF COMMITTEE,

WITH THE

Philadelphia Contributors.

Dr. *Thomas Webster, Jr., Chairman of Committee of Relief, in Account and Portsmouth*

1855.			
Aug. 15	To this sum received from Thos. Webster, Jr., General Agent of Union Steam Ship Co., being a collection made by him prior to the call for a public meeting,		$583 50
Nov. 29, "	this sum received from Block No. 1, from Vine to Arch, and from Delaware Avenue to west side of Front street.		
	Collections per A. J. Derbyshire, .	271 00	
	" Stilwell S. Bishop,.	142 50	
			413 50
Nov. 29, "	this sum received from Block No. 2, from Vine to Arch, and from Front to Schuylkill.		
	Collections per Chas. Evans and Jos. B. Myers, ...	463 50	
	" Peter Thompson, .	5 00	
	" John Agnew, . .	75 25	
	" Caleb Needles, .	30 00	
	" J. S. Natt & H. Craig,	97 00	
	" Thos. Webster, Jr.,	50 00	
	" Wharton E. Harris,	488 00	
	" Thos. J. Potts, . .	187 65	
	" C. Brazer, Alderman,	16 00	
	" J. C. Whitall, . .	47 25	
	" Caleb Clothier. . .	179 50	
			1639 15
Nov. 29, "	this sum received from Block No. 3—from Arch to Walnut and from Delaware Avenue to Front street.		
	Collections per B. B. Craycroft, .	141 00	
	" A. F. Cheesbrough,	275 00	
	" Jno. D. Taylor, .	100 00	
	" E. Morris Buckley,	171 00	
	" Thos. Webster, Jr.,	116 00	
			803 00
Nov. 29, "	this sum received from Block No 4—from Arch to North side of Market and		
			$3,439 15

with the Contributors to the Philadelphia Fund for the Relief of the Norfolk Sufferers. CR.

1855.			
Aug.	15	By Drexel & Co., Bankers' draft on R. H. Maury & Co., Richmond, remitted by Thomas Webster, Jr., General Agent Union Steamship Company, to the Mayor of Norfolk, with request to distribute $250 of same to authorities of Portsmouth, - - - - - - -	$600 00
	17	" E. W. Clark & Co. Bankers' draft on Jno. D. Gordon, Norfolk, remitted to Howard Association, Norfolk, - - - - - - -	600 00
	"	" E. W. Clark & Co., Bankers' draft on Jno. D. Gordon, Norfolk, remitted to D. D. Fiske, Mayor of Portsmouth, - - - - - -	400 00
	18	" Farmers & Mechanics' Bank's draft on Bank of Virginia, remitted to Howard Association, Norfolk, - - - - - - - - - -	600 00
	"	" Farmers & Mechanics' Bank's draft on Bank of Virginia, remitted to D. D. Fiske, Mayor of Portsmouth, - - - - - - - -	400 00
	20	" Farmers & Mechanics' Bank's draft on Bank of Virginia, remitted to Howard Association, Norfolk, - - - - - - - - - -	600 00
			$3,200 00

Dr. *Thomas Webster, Jr., in Account with the Philadelphia Contributors*

		To amount brought forward, . . .	——	$3,439 15
		from Front to Sixth street—collections per Jno. Trucks, J. B. Lippincott and J. G. Brenner, ...	1116 50	
		Collections per David Faust, .	176 00	
		" Sol. Bunn, . .	20 00	
		" James C. Hand, .	50 00	
		" Morris L. Hallowell,	300 00	
		" John Trucks, .	155 00	
		" S. Conrad & J. Patterson,	297 25	
		" David Faust & others.	326 50	
				2441 25
Nov. 29,	"	this sum received from Block No. 5—from Arch to Market and from Sixth to Schuylkill.		
		Collections per S. L. Witmer and Jas. Graham, . .	126 00	
		" A. Emerick, .	36 50	
		" J. Z. Dehaven and Wm. Nassau, Jr.,	322 25	
		" Clayton French, .	35 00	
		" Joseph Waterman,	33 60	
		" J. Thompson, Alderman.	35 00	
				588 35
Nov. 29,	"	this sum received from Block No. 6—from south side of Market street to north side of Chesnut, and from Front to Sixth street.		
		Collections per Geo. H. Martin and W. H. Inskeep,	685 00	
		" Thomas Beaver, .	145 00	
		" C. W. Wharton and C. L. Sharpless, .	357 00	
		" D. Haddock and Sol. Smith, . .	193 00	
		" Wm. S. Stewart and W. A. Drown, .	753 50	
		" Thos. Webster, Jr.,	225 00	
				2358 50
				$8,827 25

to the Fund for the Relief of the Norfolk and Portsmouth Sufferers. Cr.

		Amount brought forward.	$3,200 00
Aug.	20	By Farmers & Mechanics' Bank's draft on Bank of Virginia, remitted to D. D. Fiske, Mayor of Portsmouth, - - - - - - - - -	400 00
	21	" Farmers & Mechanics' Bank's draft on Bank of Virginia, remitted to Howard Association, Norfolk, - - - - - - - - - -	1,400 00
	"	" Farmers' & Mechanics' Bank's draft on Bank of Virginia, remitted to D. D. Fiske, Mayor of Portsmouth, - - - - - - - - -	1,000 00
	22	" E. W. Clark & Co., Bankers' draft on Jno. D. Gordon, Norfolk, remitted to Howard Association, Norfolk, - - - - - - -	600 00
	"	" E. W. Clark & Co., Bankers' draft on Jno. D. Gordon, Norfolk, remitted to D. D. Fiske, Mayor of Portsmouth, - - - - - -	400 00
	24	" Farmers & Mechanics' Bank's draft on Bank of Virginia, remitted to Howard Association, Norfolk, - - - - - - - - -	1,200 00
	"	" Farmers & Mechanics' Bank's draft on Bank of Virginia, remitted to D. D. Fiske, Mayor of Portsmouth, - - - - - - - - -	800 00
			$9,000 00

DR. *Thomas Webster, Jr., in Account with the Philadelphia Contributors*

	To amount brought forward, . .		$8,827 25
Nov. 29,	" this sum received from Block No. 7—from Walnut street to Navy Yard and Delaware Avenue to Second street.		
	Collections per J. B. Lancaster and Samuel Welsh, .	$298 00	
	" A. E. Outerbridge and S. P. Pedrick, .	75 00	
	" John Gibson, .	187 00	
	" Jos. Edwards, .	22 50	
			582 50
Nov. 29,	" This sum received from Block No. 8—from Walnut to South and from Front to Sixth streets. Collections per John H. Deihl and Wm. M. Baird, . .	492 50	
			492 50
Nov. 29,	" this sum received from Block No. 9—from Walnut to South and from Sixth street to Schuylkill.		
	Collections per Callender I. Lewis,	165 00	
	" Samuel C. Shepherd,	164 50	
	" Henry C. Blair, .	94 00	
	" James T. Shinn and S. W. Gray, .	152 00	
	" Arthur Howell, .	5 00	
	" John Goodyear, .	23 50	
	" Geo. W. Brown, .	83 00	
			687 00
Nov. 29,	" this sum received from Block No. 10—old District of Southwark.		
	Collections per Capt. David Teal, .	41 00	
	" John B. Austin,	5 00	
	" J. A. Cantrell, M.D.,	71 17	
	" A. Day, Navy Agent,	83 00	
			200 17
Nov. 29,	" this sum received from Block No. 11—from Chesnut to Walnut and from Front to Sixth streets.		
	Collections per M. Dunn (Exchange)	483 50	
	" Solomon Shepherd,	1077 09	
	" William Rice, .	235 00	
		$1,795 59	10,789 42

to the Fund for the Relief of the Norfolk and Portsmouth Sufferers. CR.

		Amount brought forward.	$9,000 00
Aug. 25	By	Cash paid Rosengarton & Son's bill for Quinine, per voucher 1, - - - - - - -	250 00
"	"	Farmers & Mechanics' Bank's draft on Bank of Virginia, remitted to Howard Association, Norfolk, - - - - - - - -	600 00
"	"	Farmers & Mechanics' Bank's draft on Bank of Virginia, remitted to D. D. Fiske, Mayor of Portsmouth, - - - - - - - -	400 00
27	"	Farmers & Mechanics' Bank's draft on Bank of Virginia, remitted to Howard Association, Norfolk, being one-half of the contribution from workmen of the Navy Yard, - - -	909 17
"	"	Farmers & Mechanics' Bank's draft on Bank of Virginia, remitted to D. D. Fiske, Mayor of Portsmouth, being one-half of the contribution of workmen at the Navy Yard, - - -	909 16
28	"	Cash paid S. A. Owen's bill for Ice Cream, per voucher 2, - - - - - - - -	24 00
29	"	Farmers & Mechanics' Bank's draft on Bank of Virginia, remitted to Howard Association, being one-half of the collection taken up in the Catholic Churches, - - - - - -	306 69
			$12,399,02

DR. *Thomas Webster, Jr., in Account with the Philadelphia Contributors*

	To amounts brought forward, . .	$1,795 59	10,789 42
	" William T. Martien,	388 00	
	" George D. Parrish,	85 00	
	" Elliston Perot, .	510 00	
	" Dr. David Jayne,	3 00	
	" S. W. Cannell,	130 00	
			2911 59
Nov. 29,	" this sum received from Block No. 12—from Chesnut to Walnut and from Sixth street to Schuylkill.		
	Collections per John West, . .	45 50	
	" A. B. Durand,	77 50	
	" A. H. Orne, .	137 00	
	" Richard Vaux, .	70 00	
	" William Parvin, Jr.,	186 00	
	" J. W. Queen . .	26 00	
	" T. W. Evans, . .	20 00	
			562 00
Nov. 29,	" this sum received from Block No. 13—from Chesnut to Market and Sixth street to Schuylkill.		
	Collections per G. C. Presbury (Girard House),	75 00	
	" S. W. Simes, .	96 00	
	" A. F. Glass (Washington House), .	158 00	
			329 00
Nov. 29,	" this sum received from Block No. 14—District of Richmond.		
	Collections per C. W. Sinnickson,	220 00	
			220 00
Nov. 29,	" this sum received from Block No. 15—old District of Kensington.		
	Collections per Hon. John Robbins, Jr., and Nathan Rowland,	208 50	
	" Theodore Birely, .	31 00	
	" James T. Sutton,	65 00	
	" Jacob Naylor, .	45 50	
	" J. P. Levy, .	32 50	
			382 50
			$15,194 51

to the Fund for the Relief of the Norfolk and Portsmouth Sufferers. Cr.

		Amount brought forward.	$12,399 02
Aug.	29	By Farmers & Mechanics' Bank's draft on Bank of Virginia, remitted to D. D. Fiske, Mayor of Portsmouth, being one-half of the collection taken up in the Catholic Churches, - - - -	306 68
	30	" Cash paid S. A. Owen's bill for Ice Cream, per voucher 3, - - - - - - - - -	30 00
	"	" Cash paid Rosengarton & Son's bill for Quinine, per voucher 5, - - - - - - - -	125 00
	31	" Cash paid R. Jennings' bill for Matresses, per voucher 5, - - - - - - - - -	66 05
	"	" Cash paid Charles Ellis' & Co.'s bill for Drugs and Medicines, per voucher 6, - - - -	451 70
	"	" Cash paid C. J. Fell & Bro.'s bill for Mustard, per voucher 7, - - - - - - - - -	72 75
	"	" Cash paid D. S. Miller, Jr.s' bill for Chloride of Lime, per voucher 8, - - - - - -	103 35
Sept.	1	" Cash paid D. & J. Noblitts' bill for Mattresses, per voucher 9, - - - - - - - - -	132 00
	2	" Cash paid Oldenberg & Taggert's bill for Shirts, per voucher 10, - - - - - - -	13 00
			$13,699 55

Dr. *Thomas Webster, Jr., in Account with the Philadelphia Contributors*

	To	amount brought forward, . . .		$15,194 51
Nov. 29,	"	this sum received from Block No. 16— old District of Northern Liberties.		
		Collections per Samuel Bolton,	$102 00	
		" A. Justice, .	5 00	
		" Wm. Esher, Jno. Kessler, Jr., S. H. Bush, Daniel M. Fox and others.	1131 47	
				1238 47
Nov. 29,	To	this sum received from Block No. 17— Old District of Spring Garden.		
		Collections per Wm. B. Thomas	85 00	
		" John Baird, .	200 00	
		" M. E. Afflick & others,	74 00	
		" John T. Taitt, .	1 00	
				$360 00
Nov. 29,	"	this sum received from Block No. 18— Old District of Moyamensing.		
		Collections per Richard George,	74 00	
				74 00
Nov. 29,	"	this sum received from Block No. 19— Old District of West Philadelphia.		
		Collections per A. B. Justice, .	40 00	
				40 00
Nov. 29,	"	this sum received from Block No. 20— Germantown and vicinity.		
		Collections per Joseph Hansberry,	49 00	
		" C. J. Wistar, Jr.,	217 75	
		" E. P. Morris, .	197 75	
		" Lloyd Mifflin, .	102 50	
		" Edwin Cope, .	62 50	
		" J. Carpenter, .	56 00	
		" G. W. Carpenter, Jr.,	40 50	
		" Messrs. Waul, Leibert and others, .	79 75	
				805 75
				$17,712 73

to the Fund for the Relief of the Norfolk and Portsmouth Sufferers. CR.

		Amount brought forward.	$13,699 55
Sept.	3	By Cash paid Isaac Jeans & Co.'s bill for Lemons, per voucher 11, - - - - - - -	134 28
	4	" Cash paid Samuel Grant, Jr.'s bill for Chloride of Lime, per voucher 12, - - - - - -	65 00
	5	" Farmers & Mechanics' Bank's draft on Bank of Virginia, remitted to Howard Association, Norfolk, - - - - - - - - - -	603 00
	"	" Farmers & Mechanics' Bank's draft on Bank of Virginia, remitted to D. D. Fiske, Mayor of Portsmouth, - - - - - - - -	402 00
	6	" Cash paid W. H. Dodge's bill for Castile Soap, per voucher 13, - - - - - - -	56 81
	"	" Cash paid Isaac S. Williams' bill for sundry articles for outfit of a nurse, per voucher 14, - -	6 33
	6	" Cash paid C. P. Elfreth's bill for Lint &c., outfit for a nurse, per voucher 15, - - - - -	3 96
	7	" Girard Bank's draft on Jno. D. Gordon, Norfolk, remitted to Howard Association, Norfolk, - -	300 00
			$15,270 93

DR. *Thomas Webster, Jr., in Account with the Philadelphia Contributors*

	To amount brought forward, ...		$17,712 73
Nov. 29,	To this sum received from Block No. 21—the Rural Districts.		
	Collections per C. Lloyd (Blue Bell),	$51 50	
	" Christopher Fallon,	50 00	
	" J. George (Belmont),	128 25	
			229 75
Nov. 29,	" this sum received from Block No. 22—At Large.		
	Collections per Wm. E. Bowen,	220 00	
			220 00
			$18,162 48

CHAIRMAN'S COLLECTIONS.

To collections made by Chairman and contributions sent to him anonymously, and otherwise,

From 17th to 27th August, inclusive	250 00	
" 28 " 31 " "	190 00	
" 1 " 5 Sept. "	194 00	
" 6 " 31 " "	773 50	
" 12 " 18 " "	380 00	
" 19 " 1 Oct. "	207 02	
" 2nd Oct. to date "	126 00	
		2120 52
To collections in company with M. L. Hallowell,		295 00

CATHOLIC CHURCHES.

Church of the Assumption, .	107 30	
St. John's, ...	227 60	
St. Mary's . . .	125 21	
St. Patrick's . . .	69 64	
St. James', . . .	41 29	
St. Malachi's, . .	32 75	
Holy Trinity, . . .	31 26	
Cathedral Chapel, . .	6 00	
St. Joseph's, . . .	86 47	
St. Philip's, . . .	54 00	
		781 52
		$3,197 04

to the Fund for the Relief of the Norfolk and Portsmouth Sufferers. Cr.

		Amount brought forward.	$15,270 93
Sept. 7	By	Girard Bank's draft on Jno. D. Gordon, Norfolk, remitted to D. D. Fiske, Mayor of Portsmouth, - - - - - - - - - -	200 00
8	"	Farmers & Mechanics' Bank's draft on Bank of Virginia, remitted to Howard Association, Norfolk, - - - - - - - - -	1005 00
"	"	Farmers & Mechanics' Bank's draft on Bank of Virginia, remitted to D. D. Fiske, Mayor of Portsmouth, - - - - - - - -	502 50
"	"	Cash paid W. Mason's bill for Lime Juice, voucher 16, - - - - - - - - . -	66 80
"	"	Cash paid Rosengarton & Son's bill for Quinine, per voucher 17, - - - - - - -	125 00
"	"	Cash paid X. Bazin's bill for Bay Rum, Aromatic Vinegar and Cologne Water, per voucher 18, -	112 00
"	"	Cash paid S. A. Owen's bill for Ice Cream, per voucher 19, - - - - - - - - -	12 00
11	"	Farmers & Mechanics' Bank's draft on Bank of Virginia, remitted to Howard Association, Norfolk, - - - - - -	3000 00
			$20,294 23

DR. *Thomas Webster, Jr., in Account with the Philadelphia Contributors*

To amount brought forward,		———	$18,162 48
Chairman's Statement brought forward, ...		3,197 04	

PRESBYTERIAN CHURCHES.

Central Presbyterian Church, Coates street, . . .	50 00		
Church at Frankford, . .	64 06		
Tenth, Rev. Mr. Boardman, .	370 00		
Sixth, Rev. J. H. Jones, .	100 37		
First, at Germantown, per C. J. Wistar, Chairman, . .	142 00		
Church at Doylestown, Bucks Co.,	55 00		
Church at Roxborough, . .	10 88		
	———	792 31	

PROTESTANT EPISCOPAL CHURCHES.

All Saints, Lower Dublin—prior to Bishop Potter's Letter, . .	50 00		
" " Additional,	26 00		
Holy Trinity, Westchester—prior to Bishop Potter's Letter, .	31 50		
" " Additional,	10 00		
St. Andrew's per Messrs. Robbins & Coffin,	94 50		
[From members thereof no collection taken up.]			
St. John's, Norristown, . .	75 00		
St. Matthew's, Francisville, .	63 53		
St. Peter's, . .	292 86		
St. Luke's, ...	417 69		
St. Paul's, . .	300 00		
St. Jame's, ...	249 50		
Mission Chapel, St. Luke's, Germantown, . . .	8 00		
Epiphany, . . .	537 00		
St. James the Less, .	63 30		
St. Andrew's, Mantuaville, .	23 50		
Church of the Advent, .	130 78		
	$2,373 16	$3,989 35	$18,162 48

to the Fund for the Relief of the Norfolk and Portsmouth Sufferers. Cr.

	To amount brought forward, ...	$20,294 23
Sept. 11,	By Farmers and Mechanics' Bank's draft on Bank of Virginia, remitted to D. D. Fiske, Mayor of Portsmouth, . . .	2,000 00
	" Cashpaid Harris & Heyls, bill for Wines and Brandy, per voucher 20, . . .	46 00
12,	" Farmers and Mechanics' Bank's draft on Bank of Virginia, remitted to D. D. Fiske, Mayor of Portsmouth, with a request to forward same to Suffolk, in case the report that the fever had broke out in that town should prove true; if unfounded, to apply it to wants of Portsmouth. The latter was done.	500 00
		$22,840 23

Dr. *Thomas Webster, Jr., in Account with the Philadelphia Contributors*

To amount brought forward, . . .			$18,162 48
Chairman's Statement, continued,—			
Amount brought forward, .		$3,989 35	
Prot. Episcopal Churches, continued—			
Amount brought over,	$2,373 16		
Church of the Nativity, .	85 50		
Grace Church, . .	290 18		
St. James, Kingsessing,	156 57		
St. Luke's, Germantown, .	150 77		
All Saints', . . .	30 01		
Gloria Dei, . . .	59 00		
Church of the Atonement,. .	189 79		
Trinity, Southwark, .	148 50		
Church of the Messiah, Richmond,	18 00		
St. Paul's, Chesnut Hill, .	81 00		
St. Mark's, . . .	200 00		
St. Paul's, Bloomsburg, .	10 00		
Church of the Evangelist, .	31 00		
St. Mary's, West Philadelphia,	87 00		
Church of the Mediator, .	20 20		
Emanuel, Kensington, .	50 25		
Calvary Church or Bishop White Chapel, ...	14 50		
Church of the Redemption, .	13 65		
Zion [Mission], Kensington, .	7 00		
Grace Church, Honesdale, .	20 81		
St. Mark's, Frankford, . .	102 69		
St. John's, Northern Liberties,	42 17		
St. David's, Manayunk, . .	108 50		
Emanuel, Holmesburg, .	101 97		
Church of the Ascension, .	64 03		
St. Philip's, . . .	255 00		
Church of the Saviour, West Phila.	34 38		
Ascension, Claymont, Delaware Co.,	21 00		
Christ Church, Germantown,	110 50		
St. John's, Bellefonte, Centre Co.,	6 00		
Calvary, Rockdale, Delaware Co.,	10 00		
St. John's " " .	5 00		
Christ Church, Torresdale, .	30 00		
	$4,928 13	$3,989 35	$18,162 48

to the Fund for the Relief of the Norfolk and Portsmouth Sufferers. Cr.

	Amount brought forward, ...	22,840 23
14,	" Cash handed to the Widow of H. Spriggman, a volunteer Nurse, who returned and died here, per voucher 20¼, . . .	30 00
14,	" Farmers and Mechanics' Bank's draft on Bank of Virginia, remitted to Howard Association, Norfolk, (making a total in cash, up to this date, $14,000), . .	1,926 15
	" Farmers and Mechanics' Bank, draft on Bank of Virginia, remitted to D. D. Fiske, Mayor of Portsmouth, (making a total in cash, up to this date, of $10,000), . .	1,129 65
15,	" Cash advanced up to this date, in sums of five and ten dollars, to seventy-eight persons, Doctors, Druggists, Nurses, volunteers to aid sufferers, for incidental and travelling expenses, ...	709 50
		$26,635 53

Dr. *Thomas Webster, Jr., in Account with the Philadelphia Contributors*

To amount brought forward, ...			$18,162 48
Chairman's Statement, continued—			
Amount brought forward, . .		$3,989 35	
Prot. Episcopal Churches, continued—			
Amount brought over,	4,928 13		
Trinity, Oxford, Phila. Co.,	300 50		
Trinity, Washington, Pa. .	5 00		
St. Martin's, Marcus Hook,	31 13		
Christ Church, . .	231 42		
St. Thomas, Whitemarsh, .	53 00		
St. Bartholomew's, . .	20 00		
St. Paul's, Chester, . .	42 00		
Christ Church, Leacock, Lancaster Co.,	5 00		
St. Stephen's, Wilkesbarre, .	97 00		
Church of the Redeemer, .	25 25		
St. James, Perkiomen, .	10 78		
Union, Lower Providence, Montgomery County, . .	9 45		
St. Mark's, Chester, .	15 00		
St. Johns', Pequa, Lancaster Co.,	5 00		
Swede's Church, Upper Merion,	38 00		
St. John's Pequa, per *Penna. Inquirer* Office, . .	18 50		
All Saints' Paradise. . .	14 00		
		5849 16	
BAPTIST CHURCHES.			
First Baptist Church, .	156 50		
Calvary " Second Ward,	141 80		
First " Bristol,	28 00		
Fifth " . .	44 47		
		370 77	
HEBREW CHURCHES, &c.			
Portuguese Jewish Congregation,	100 00		
German Hebrew Congregation,	25 00		
Hebrew Literary Association,	10 00		
Benai Israel, . .	25 00		
		160 00	
MORAVIAN CHURCH, . .		70 69	
		$10,439 97	$18,162 48

to the Fund for the Relief of the Norfolk and Portsmouth Sufferers. Cr

	Amount brought forward, ...			$26,635 53
	" Cash paid Sickle & Jones for printing bills, "Contributions, &c., received here," per voucher 21, ...			2 50
Sept. 15,	By Cash paid J. R. Luce, Live Chickens,	per vch'r	22,	165 25
"	" R. McElroy, Fresh Butter	"	23,	66 50
"	" C. H. Cummings, Hay,	"	24,	75 09
"	" John McQuaid, Ice Cream,	"	25,	75 00
"	" Thomas Ramsey, Bread,	"	26,	22 11
"	" Charles Ellis & Co., Medicines,	"	27,	190 00
"	" E. G. Whitman, Guava Jelly,	"	28,	13 50
"	" Frederick Brown, Ginger,	"	29,	10 00
"	" L. W. Glenn & Co., Aromatic Vinegar, . . .	"	30,	5 70
				$27,261 18

DR. *Thomas Webster, Jr., in Account with the Philadelphia Contributors*

Amount brought forward, . . .			$18,162 48
Chairman's Statement continued—			
Amount brought forward, .		$10,439 97	
PROTESTANT ASSOCIATIONS.			
Joshua Lodge, No. 14, American Protestants, ...	20 00		
Mount Olive Lodge, No. 52, American Protestants, ...	14 62		
Liberty Lodge, No. 9, American Protestants, ...	56 00		
		90 62	
FROM WORKSHOPS, FACTORIES, &c.			
Master Workmen, Mechanics, and Laborers of Navy Yard—being one day's pay — per Francis Grice, Naval Constructor,	$1,855 83		
A few German Mechanics, .	8 25		
Workmen in B. Elsler's Turner Shop, ...	7 50		
Workmen in D. G. Wilson & Co.'s Wheelwright and Blacksmith Shop, ...	132 50		
Workmen in Geo. Adler's Morocco Factory, ...	51 16		
Workmen in M. W. Baldwin & Co.'s Locomotive Engine Works,	150 97		
Men and Boys in employ of Knickerbocker Ice Company, .	50 00		
Letter Carriers in U. S. Post Office,	77 00		
Clerks, and Attachees, of Sheriff's Office, ...	75 00		
One day's wages of Workmen at the Marble and Mahogany Establishment of Lewis Thompson & Co., ...	126 24		
	$2,534 45	$10,530 59	$18,162 48

to the Fund for the Relief of the Norfolk and Portsmouth Sufferers. Cr.

Amount brought forward, . . .				$27,261 18
Sept. By cash paid	R. McElroy, Fresh Butter,	"	31,	110 40
" "	J. R. Luce, Live Chickens,	"	32,	174 50
" "	J. H. Peters & Co., Arom. Vin.,	"	33,	4 59
" "	Sharpless Brothers, Merino for a Nurse, . . .	"	34,	6 00
" "	Mercer & Antelo, Hams,	"	35,	263 10
" "	McCutcheon & Collins, Hams,	"	36,	17 87
" "	G. P. Green, for Toasted Bread,	"	37,	91 62
" "	Thomas Ramsey, Bread,	"	38,	46 52
" "	S. A. Owens, Ice Cream,	"	39,	10 50
" "	Joseph M. Oliver, Guava Jelly,	"	40,	18 87
" "	J. F. Cake, Roasted and Ground Coffee, . . .	"	41,	55 00
				$28,060 15

Dr. *Thomas Webster, Jr., in Account with the Philadelphia Contributors*

Amount brought forward, ...			$18,162 48
Chairman's Statement continued—			
Amount brought forward, . .		$10,530 59	
Workshops, Factories, &c., continued—			
Amount brought over, .	$2,534 45		
Ladies employed at Brook, Brothers & Co., No. 91 N. Third Street,	20 00		
Workmen employed by Reanny, Neaffie & Co., at Penn Iron Works, ...	113 75		
Men and Boys employed at Miles B. Espy's Pickling Establishment, ...	22 55		
Workmen employed at S. Merrick & Son's Works, Southwark, .	310 22		
Workmen in the employ of N. Coleman & Son, Wagon Builders, Kensington, ...	50 00		
Clerks and Messengers in U. S. Post Office, ...	123 00		
Operatives in the Factory of D. Milne & Son, . . .	100 00		
Men employed by Bancroft, Sellers & Co., Machinists, . .	44 50		
Employees of the Publishing House of J. B. Lippincott & Co., .	200 50		
Workmen at P. S. Duval & Co.'s Lithographic Establishment,	52 25		
Young Men attached to No. 98 Market Street, . . .	15 00		
Workmen employed at Neall, Mathews & Co., Bush Hill Iron Works, ...	120 00		
Workmen in C. C. & P. Warner's Watch Case Factory, . .	25 00		
Workmen in Chas. Williams' Marble Paper Factory, . . .	6 00		
Police Officers of 4th Ward, .	30 00		
Workmen employed by Cornelius & Baker, ...	632 50		
Workmen in William Hammond's Bakery, ...	3 00		
	$4,402 72	$10,530 59	$18,162 48

to the Fund for the Relief of the Norfolk and Portsmouth Sufferers. Cr.

Amount brought forward, ...		$28,060 15
By cash paid Lewis & Co., Blankets,	per voucher 42,	520 81
" " J. Palmer & Co., Lard,	" 43,	81 63
" " Rand & Chenoweth, Medicines,	" 44,	96 00
" Cash paid Farmers and Mechanics' Bank, draft on Bank of Virginia, remitted to Howard Association, Norfolk, being three-fifths of the Reading contribution, with exchange added, ...		453 33
" Farmers and Mechanics' Bank's draft on Bank of Virginia, remitted to Holt Wilson, Treasurer of Sanitary Committee of Portsmouth, being two-fifths of the Reading contribution, with exchange added, .		302 21
By cash paid Roussel & Parsons, for Mineral Water, .	per voucher 45,	280 00
		$29,794 13

Dr. *Thomas Webster, Jr., in Account with the Philadelphia Contributors*

Amount brought forward, . .			$18,162 48
Chairman's Statement continued—			
Amount brought forward, . .		$10,530 59	
Workshops, Factories, &c., continued—			
Amount brought forward,	$4,402 72		
Workmen in Colwell & Co.'s Conshohocken Works, . .	82 38		
Workmen in William D. Rodgers' Carriage Factory, . . .	112 00		
Workmen of Dentz & Wensell, Jewelers.	6 75		
Workmen in I. P. Morris & Co.'s Foundry and Works at Port Richmond, ...	100 75		
Employees in Dental Manufactory of Jones, White & McCurdy,	50 00		
Printers and others connected with the Pennsylvania Inquirer, .	100 00		
Workmen in G. W. Simons' Gold Thimble and Pencil Factory,	30 00		
Workmen at Walter Cresson's, .	50 00		
Workmen in S. P. Opdike's Gold Chain Factory, . . .	15 00		
Employees in the Lithographic Establishment of Walters & McGuigans, ...	54 50		
Workmen at the Dyottville Glass Works, per J. M. Benners, .	47 50		
Hands employed in Geo. J. Weaver & Co.'s Rope Walk and Jenny House, ...	101 48		
Hands employed in H. B. Odiorne's Machine Sewing Establishment,	26 00		
Operatives in Thomas Drake's Cotton and Woollen Mills, . .	70 00		
Operatives in the employ of Wakefield Manufacturing Company, per C. J. Wistar, Jr., . .	45 50		
Hands employed by W. Allen, per C. J. Wistar, . . .	16 00		
	$5,310 58	$10,530 59	$18,162 48

to the Fund for the Relief of the Norfolk and Portsmouth Sufferers. Cr.

Amount brought forward, . . .		$29,794	13
By cash paid John Garrison & Co., Claret,	vchr. 45½,	180	75
" " Henry Apple, for a Half-barrel,	" 36,	1	50
" " T. H. Jacobs & Co., Wines and Brandies, . . .	" 47,	814	70
" " S. C. Sheppard, Citrate of Magnesia, ...	" 48,	36	75
' " Rosengarten & Co., Quinine and Sulphate of Morphia, .	" 49,	67	00
" " Atlee & Evans, Oranges,	" 50,	78	75
" " Bond & Denklais, Tea	" 51,	199	29
" " Ellwood Matlacks, Boys' Clothing, . . .	" 52,	315	00
" " Wm. Murtha, Stockings,	" 53,	62	50
		$31,550	37

Dr. *Thomas Webster, Jr., in Account with the Philadelphia Contributors*

To amount brought forward, . . .			$18,162 48
Chairman's Statement continued—			
Amount brought forward, .		$10,530 59	
Workshops, Factories, &c., continued—			
Amount brought forward, .	$5,310 58		
Attachees and Employees of Haley, Ware & Co.'s Cottage Furniture Manufactory, . . .	85 25		
Stone Cutters in employ of S. F. Prince, ...	26 00		
Workmen in employ of E. & G. Brooke, Birdsboro', Berks Co.,	45 00		
Operatives in Cotton and Woollen Mills of Wm. Divine, . .	97 52		
Men employed at Gas Works, Market Street, Schuylkill, . .	195 00		
Men employed at Gas Office, Seventh Street, ...	40 00		
Cutters at U. S. Arsenal, . .	9 00		
Men employed by Military Storekeeper, ...	105 82		
Clerks in "Office of Army and Clothing Equipage," . .	8 50		
Workmen in B. D. Stewart's Morocco Factory, . . .	35 00		
Employees of Pennsylvania Railroad Company, at West Philadelphia, ...	117 51		
Workmen at James and John Hunter's Hyde Part Print Works, in Belmont District, . . .	59 30		
A few of the Hands employed at Penn Stove Works, . .	18 50		
Workmen at E. P. Molineaux's Shoe Factory, . . .	14 25		
Workmen at Gas Works, Point Breeze, ...	200 62		
U. S. Mint, per Michael Dunn,	48 75		
Ericsson Steamboat Line, .	50 00		
Attachees of Drexel & Co., Bankers,	50 00		
	$6,516 60	$10,530 59	$18,162 48

to the Fund for the Relief of the Norfolk and Portsmouth Sufferers. CR.

Amount brought forward, ...			$31,550 37
By cash paid R. McElroy, Butter,	"	54,	103 30
" " Joseph Luce, Live Chickens,	"	55,	164 00
" " Allen & Hugels, Sago and Farina,	"	56,	59 67
" " Van Brunt, Tripler & Combs, Hams and Tongues,	"	57,	239 78
" " R. D. Clifton and P. McCormack, for Clothing for a person from Portsmouth, found suffering from an attack of the Fever in our streets, taken to City Hospital and discharged cured, . . .	"	58,	11 00
" Advanced to same person to enable him to get to Boston to his family,	"	59,	6 00
" Paid S. J. Moore, for Leeches,	"	60,	22 00
" " X. Bazin, Aromatic Vinegar and Cologne, . .	"	61,	51 50
			$32,207 62

DR. *Thomas Webster, Jr., in Account with the Philadelphia Contributors*

Amount brought forward, . .			$18,162 48
Chairman's Statement continued—			
Amount brought forward, . .		$10,530 59	
*Workshops, Factories, &c., continued—			
Amount brought forward, .	6,516 60		
Employees in Freight Depot of Reading Railroad, . .	55 00		
Employees of L. Johnson & Co., Type and Stereotype Foundry,	150 00		
Employees of Fritz, Hendry & Co.,	50 00		
Laborers on Section 19, 20, and 21, of Lebanon Valley Railroad,	66 50		
Workmen of Bushnell & Tull,	27 00		
Workmen in W. E. Morgan's Spectacle Factory, . . .	15 00	6,880 10	
FIREMEN.			
Northern Liberties Hose Company, per Michael Dunn, of the Exchange, ...	80 10		
Schuylkill Hose Company, . .	50 00		
Members of Diligent Engine Co.,	100 00	230 10	
SONS OF TEMPERANCE.			
Fraternal Division, No. 49, .	10 00		
Division, No. 3, Germantown, . . .	10 00	20 00	
"WILLIAM HANNING'S CITY LAGER BEER SALOON," one day's receipts thereof, ...		120 00	
FRIENDSHIP UNION, No. 4, "United Order of Brothers and Sisters,"		30 00	
		$17,810 79	$18,162 48

* $25 was received through the Committee collecting in Northern Liberties, from Workmen employed at Daniel Ereland's Morocco Factory, and has been credited in collections of Block 16.

to the Fund for the Relief of the Norfolk and Portsmouth Sufferers. Cr.

Amount brought forward, . . .		$32,207 62
By cash paid J. C. Wilson & Co., for Provisions bought in Baltimore by Captain Nathan Thompson, Steward of the Committee, and Travelling Agent, to relieve the wants of a colony of refugees, whom he found encamped below Norfolk, near Tanner's Creek, suffering for the commonest necessities of life,	" 62,	178 76
By cash paid Isaac Jeanes & Co, Lemons,	" 63,	260 63
" " Joseph B. Bussier, Preserved Ginger and Bay Rum,	" 64,	104 67
" " S. Morris Waln & Co., East India Ale, . . .	" 65,	29 56
		$32,781 24

DR. *Thomas Webster, Jr., in Account with the Philadelphia Contributors*

Amount brought forward, . .		———	$18,162 48
Chairman's Statement continued—			
Amount brought forward, . .		$17,810 79	
SHAWNEE TRIBE, No. —, Improved Order of Red Men, . . .		30 00	
DEBORAH FRANKLIN COUNCIL, No. 2, Daughters of America, ...		10 00	
ROTTEK GROVE, UNITED ANCIENT ORDER OF DRUIDS, . .		15 00	
ARTILLERY CORPS, WASHINGTON GRAYS, ...		50 00	

AMUSEMENTS.

Proceeds of a Concert at Parkinson's Garden, September 10th,	509 06		
Managers, Actors, and Attachees of Arch Street Theatre, . .	200 00		
Proceeds of a Benefit at City Museum, Sept. —, . . .	140 00		
Proceeds of a Lecture by Professor Whitaker, on the Beautiful, at West Philadelphia, . .	83 50		
Proceeds of Melon Street Soiree,	1 50		
Proceeds of a Concert of Maennerchor and Concordia Vocal Societies, on Sept. —, . . .	105 87		
	———	1,039 93	

INDEPENDENT ORDER OF ODD FELLOWS.

Columbia Lodge,	No. 36,	25 00		
Empire "	" 104,	13 00		
Harmony "	" 16,	50 00		
Philomathean Lodge,	" 10,	20 00		
Wayne "	" 3,	25 00		
Palestine "	" 271,	10 00		
Gen. Warren "	" 126,	20 00		
Commercial "	" 20,	20 00		
		———	———	———
		$183 00	$18,955 72	$18,162 48

to the Fund for the Relief of the Norfolk and Portsmouth Sufferers. CR.

Amount brought forward, ...			$32,781 24
By cash paid W. Maddock, Fine Groceries,	vchr.	66,	198 75
" " Wm. Hannings, Cheese,	"	67,	4 25
" " Miles B. Espy, Currant Jelly,	"	68,	97 00
" " Oldenberg & Taggert, Shirts and Drawers, . .	"	69,	60 12
" " Roussel & Parsons, Mineral Water, . . .	"	70,	15 00
" " W. A. & L. Shumways, Shoes,	"	71,	431 50
" " David S. Brown & Co., Blankets and Flannels, . .	"	72,	518 19
" " David S. Brown & Co., Muslin,	"	73,	43 02
" " Merino & Yeaton, Brown Stout,	"	74,	42 00
" " Atlee & Evans, Lemons and Oranges, . . .	"	75,	139 00
			$34,330 07

DR. *Thomas Webster, Jr., in Account with the Philadelphia Contributors*

Amount brought forward, .			$18,162 48
Chairman's Statement continued—			
Amount brought forward, . .		$18,955 72	
Independent Order of Odd Fellows, continued—			
Amount brought forward, .	$183 00		
Richmond " " 240,	10 00		
Temple of Honor, " 3,	10 00		
Justice Lodge, " 186,	10 00		
Metropolitan Lodge, " 150,	25 00		
Enterprise " " 201,	25 00		
Purity, " " 325,	25 00		
A Lodge which desires to be unknown, ...	20 00		
Roxborough Lodge, No. —,	10 00		
American Star Lodge, " —,	30 00		
Purity Lodge, left at Bulletin Office, ...	5 00		
Fredonia Lodge, No. 145,	25 00		
Veritas " " 443,	20 00		
Iroquois " " 508,	10 00		
Schiller, " " 95,	15 00		
Roxborough Encampment, " 66,	10 00		
Orphans' Rest Lodge, " 132, Delaware County, .	10 00		
Lewisburg Lodge, " —,	11 00		
Pocahontas " " 316,	67 50		
Farmers and Mechanics' Lodge, ... " 185,	5 00		
Montgomery Lodge, " 57,	15 00		
Norristown Encampment, " 37,	35 00		
Coaquanock Lodge, " 463,	20 00		
Grace Lodge, (Orwigsburg)" 157,	10 00		
Southwark Lodge, " 146,	10 00		
Excelsior " " 46,	20 00		
Protection " " —,	10 00		
Mystic "(Holmesb'g)" —,	8 00		
Fraternal " " —,	10 00		
Templar " " 258.	10 00		
United States " " 34,	15 00		
Moyamensing Lodge, " 330,	10 00		
Philanthropic " " 15,	20 00		
	$719 50	$18,955 72	$18,162 48

to the Fund for the Relief of the Norfolk and Portsmouth Sufferers. Cr.

Amount brought forward, . . .			$34,330 07
By cash paid Sharpless & Bro., Black Prints,	vchr.	76,	29 25
" " Union Benevolent Society, for Female Garments,	"	77,	119 62
" " G. W. Glenn & Co., Aromatic Vinegar, . . .	"	78,	9 50
" " E. C. Knight & Co., Barley,	"	79,	11 57
" " Thomas Pratt, Ice Cream,	"	80,	62 50
" " William Murtha, Stockings,	"	81,	161 38
Nov. 19, By Cash paid Harris & Heyls, Raspberry Vinegar, ...	"	82,	21 80
" " Ricketts & Watson, Crackers,	"	83,	13 28
" " J. W. Evans, Dress for a Nurse,	"	84,	2 50
" " Durand & Tourtelot, Aromatic Vinegar, . . .	"	85,	3 36
			$34,764 83

Dr. *Thomas Webster, Jr., in Account with the Philadelphia Contributors*

Amount brought forward, . .			$18,162 48
Chairman's Statement continued—			
Amount brought forward, . .		$18,955 72	
Independent Order of Odd Fellows, continued—			
Amount brought forward, .	$719 50		
Warren Lodge, No. —,	10 00		
Hope " " 93,	10 00		
Wildey Lodge, (Frankford) " 12,	25 00		
		764 50	
CORPORATIONS—(In part only, many contributions having gone to credit of the Blocks in which they were collected.)			
Board of Brokers, . . .	100 00		
Philadelphia, Baltimore, and Wilmington Railroad Company, .	100 00		
Franklin Fire Insurance Co., .	200 00		
Directors of Camden and Amboy Railroad Company, . .	200 00		
		600 00	

THROUGH NEWSPAPERS.

Left at Office of North American,	176 00		
" " Ledger, . .	12 75		
" " Bulletin, . .	52 00		
" " Penna. Inquirer,	1,132 50		
		1,373 75	

Other sums were also left at the above offices, but being from Churches, Schools, Workshops, and Brotherhoods, are acknowledged under their appropriate heads.

CONCESSIONS ON BILLS.

To this amount given by Tradesmen, when being paid their bills, independent of discount, .		117 08	
		$21,811 05	$18,162 48

to the Fund for the Relief of the Norfolk and Portsmouth Sufferers. CR.

Amount brought forward.		$34,764 83	
By cash paid T. S. Jacobs & Co., Wines, per vchr.	86,		67 00
" " Dulles, Earle & Cope, Sponges,	" 87,		22 50
" " David Woelper, Beef,	" 88,		77 18
" " C. J. Fell & Brother, Mustard,	" 89,		78 00
" " Robert Newlin, Brown Stout,	" 90,		200 00
" " Ricketts & Watson, Crackers,	" 91,		65 00
" " Allen Cuthbert, Tea,	" 92,		28 00
" " Harris & Heyls, Groceries,	" 93,		93 00
" " Jacob Snider, Wines,	" 94,		90 00
" " Grant & Twells, Broma,	" 95,		36 50
" " J. S. Bloodgood, Wine,	" 95½,		30 00

$35,552 01

Dr. *Thomas Webster, Jr., in Account with the Philadelphia Contributors*

Amount brought over, . .			$18,162 48
Chairman's Statement continued—			
Amount brought over, . .		$21,811 05	
EXCHANGE.			
To 1 per cent. difference on this amount, $600, bought of Drexel & Co, ...	6 00		
To ½ per cent. difference on this amount, $2000, bought of E. W. Clark & Co., ...	10 00		
To 1 per cent. difference on this amount, $9,807, bought of Farmers and Mechanics' Bank, .	98 07		
To ½ per cent. difference on this amount, $11,056, bought of Farmers and Mechanics' Bank, .	55 28		
To ½ per cent. difference on this amount, $500, bought of Girard Bank, ...	2 50		
To ½ per cent. discount and Exchange on Check in Savings Bank at Portsmouth, cashed for a citizen of that place. . .	1 50		
		173 35	
FROM SCHOOLS AND CHILDREN.			
Ringgold Grammar School, Moyamensing, ...	13 24		
Madison Grammar Schools, Girls' department, ...	39 00		
A Lad of St. Luke's Sunday School,	25		
Students of St. Joseph's, Willing's Alley, ...	30 00		
Boys' Grammar School, Zane St.,	60 83		
" " " New St.,	36 54		
Pupils of Mrs. Durnett's private School, 21 Parrish Street, .	2 00		
Boys of Jefferson Grammar School,	56 55		
Girls of " " "	40 75		
Boys of Madison " "	40 00		
	$319 16	$21,984 40	$18,162 48

	Amount brought over, ...	$35,552 01
Nov.	To cash left with Howard Association, Norfolk, by Dr. A. B. Campbell, being the contribution of a citizen of Philadelphia, ...	50 00
	" Cash expended by Capt. Nathan Thompson, Steward and Traveling Agent, being his disbursements for porterage, on merchandise, from depot at Baltimore, to Norfolk steamboat, and various incidental expenses, including bedding bought for the refugees at Tanner's Creek per voucher 96, . . .	61 00
	" Cash paid to Families of deceased volunteers, per vouchers 97 to 99, . .	150 00
	" Cash paid to the Widow and five children of a Norfolk citizen, on recommendation of the Norfolk Committee, per voucher 100, ...	50 00
		$35,863 01

Dr. *Thomas Webster, Jr., in Account with the Philadelphia Contributors*

Amount brought forward, .			$18,162 48
Chairman's Statement continued—			
Amount brought forward, .		$21,984 40	
From Schools and Children continued—			
Amount brought forward,	$319 16		
Proceeds of a Fair conducted by Children, No. 106, N. Sixth St.,	21 29		
Six little girls, ...	2 00		
Cadets of Temperance, Elm Tree Section, No. 29, . . .	7 00		
Proceeds of a Fair conducted by children at M. Hallowell's, near Germantown, ...	17 00		
Boys of Monroe Grammar School,	39 00		
Young Ladies of Aston Ridge Seminary, ...	18 87		
A Lad's Savings, . . .	7 00		
A Sunday School Class of Church of Nativity, ...	2 00		
Girls of Locust street Grammar School, ...	28 12		
Boys of Locust street Grammar School, ...	73 00		
Sunday School of Christ Church,	37 89		
M. for the Orphans, . . .	5 00		
Rutledge Boys' School, Seventh street below Germantown Road,	26 25		
Rutledge Girls' School, Seventh street below Germantown Road,	32 57		
Walnut street Old School, first department, ...	12 00		
Walnut street Old School, Secondary Department, . . .	8 00		
Girls of same School 200 Garments, materials procured, cut out and made up by them.			
Rowlandville Public School, 22d Section, ...	19 25		
Girls of Hancock Grammar School,	45 50		
Boys of " "	54 00		
	$774 90	21,984 40	18,162 48

the Fund for the Relief of the Norfolk and Portsmouth Sufferers. Cr.

Amount brought forward, . . .	$35,863 01
" Cash paid to man and wife, of Norfolk, in distress here, on recommendation, &c., per voucher 101, ...	10 00
" Cash paid to a citizen of Portsmouth, in distress here, on recommendation, &c., per voucher 102.	10 00
" Cash expended for Testimonials to Doctors, Druggists, and Nurses per vouchers 103 to 121, ...	1,692 00
" Cash sent to Howard Association, to defray expenses of sending on an orphan to his relatives in this city, . .	10 00
	$37,585 01

Dr. *Thomas Webster, Jr., in Account with the Philadelphia Contributors*

Amount brought forward, .			$18,162 48
Chairman's statement continued—			
Amount brought forward, .		$21,984 40	
From Schools and Children continued—			
Amount brought forward, .	$774 90		
Sabbath School of 10th Baptist Church, ...	12 50		
Roberts' Primary School, 22d Section, ...	24 50		
Pupils of Spring Garden Academy, 8th and Buttonwood streets, .	14 50		
Sabbath Schools of Central Presbyterian Church, . . .	46 50		
Pupils of N. W. Grammar School,	23 25		
" " "	53 00		
W. W. for the Orphans, . .	10 00		
Norristown Girls' Grammar School, And 100 Garments.	16 00		
Deal Street Primary School, Port Richmond, ...	8 00		
A Little Boy, ...	5 00		
Ringgold Grammar School, .	27 00		
Franklin School, Rural Districts, First Ward, ...	2 75		
A School, ...	11 00		
Bible Class, 10th Baptist Church,	2 00		
Sabbath School, 2d Associate Presbyterian Church Kensington,	27 41		
Woodville Presbyterian Sabbath School, ...	3 50		
Girls of S. E. Grammar School, 118 garments, materials purchased, cut out and made up by them.	———	1,061 81	

PENNSYLVANIA.

A Citizen of Pottstown, . .	$5 00		
Citizens of Pottsville, per . .	108 00		
A Citizen of Lebanon, . .	30 00		
" Friendsville, . .	5 00		
	$148 00	23,046 21	18,162 48

	Amount brought forward, . . .		$37,585 01
	EXPENSES.		
Nov.	To Cash paid for Telegraphing, . . .	4 57	
	" Cash paid for postage on Newspapers sent to Doctors, &c., ...	1 75	
	" Cash paid Geo. W. Grice, (Thomas Webster, Jr.'s Clerk,) bill for Stationery, Envelopes, Postage stamps, and sundry small items $5, per voucher 122, .	30 25	
	" Cash paid sundry porterages on Medicines, Provisions, and Merchandise, to Depot at Broad and Prime Streets,	16 50	
	" Cash paid Cab hire, six times, for Chairman, to Depot at Broad and Prime Sts.,	6 00	
		$59 07	$37,585 01

DR. *Thomas Webster, Jr., in Account with the Philadelphia Contributors*

Amount brought forward, .				$18,162 48
Chairman's statement continued—				
Amount brought forward, .			$23,046 21	
Pennsylvania continued—				
Amount brought forward, .		$148 00		
Citizens of Shippensburg, .		100 00		
R. K. of Minersville, per Harris & Heyl, ...		50 00		
Citizens of Bellefonte, . .		277 50		
A Citizen of Sunbury, . .		25 00		
Citizens of Hollidaysburg, .		178 63		
" West Chester and its vicinity, ...		270 89		
Citizens of Hollidaysburg, .		21 00		
" Reading, per Wm. M. Baird, Mayor, remitted specially as directed,	$751 78			
Exchange on same, .	3 76	755 54		
Citizens of Bethlehem, Shinnersville and Freemansburg, .		55 25		
"Village Record," office Westchester, ...		31 25		
Ladies of Bethlehem, . .		245 00		
Citizens of Bristol, . . .		124 34		
Citizens of Lower Merion, Montgomery Co., ...		82 90		
Citizens of Paradise, Lancaster Co.,		50 00		
			2,415 30	
NEW JERSEY.				
Mount Holly Lodge, No. 19, I. O. O. F., ...		$5 00		
Camden Council, No. 2, U. N. A.,		25 00		
Citizens of Swedesboro, . .		20 00		
" Bridgeton, . .		500 00		
First Baptist Church, Camden, .		55 00		
Citizens of Burlington, . .		60 00		
Columbus Presbyterian Church,		12 52		
Prost. Episcopal Church, Mt. Holly,		75 00		
		$752 52	25,461 51	18,162 48

to the Fund for the Relief of the Norfolk and Portsmouth Sufferers. CR.

Amount brought over, ...			$37,585 01
Expenses Continued—			
Amount brought over,		59 07	
" Cash paid Hogan & Bechtel, bill for Collection Books, Paper, Stationery, &c.. per voucher 123, ...		32 89	
" S. Shepherd, (per voucher 124,) bill, viz:			
For Contribution Boxes, .	2 50		
Cab hire to Agricultural Fair,	1 50		
Delivering Bishop Potter's Letter to Churches, . . .	5 00		
Dispatch Stamps, . .	1 10		
Wm. Maas, for Printing, .	2 50		
		12 60	
" Cash paid Wharton E. Harris, for Printing Circulars for Block 2, per vchr. 125,		7 00	
" Cash paid John Kessler, Jr., for Printing Circulars for Block 16, per voucher 126,		7 00	
		$118 56	37,585 01

Dr. *Thomas Webster, Jr., in Account with the Philadelphia Contributors*

Amount brought forward, .			$18,162 48
Chairman's statement continued—			
Amount brought forward, .		$25,461 21	
New Jersey continued—			
Amount brought forward, .	$752 52		
Baptist Church, Mount Holly, .	8 11		
Methodist Church, " .	22 15		
Presbyterian Church, " .	33 02		
Mount Holly Beneficial Society,	25 00		
Citizens of Woodbury and vicinity, for Orphans, ...	158 25		
St. John's Church, Salem, . .	130 00		
Presbyterian Church, Salem, .	110 00		
Christ Church, Woodbury, .	12 00		
Upper Township, Cape May Co.,	20 00		
St. Paul's Church, Camden, .	111 10		
Methodist Church, " .	52 88		
Presbyterian Church, additional,	1 50		
Citizens of Cape May Court House,	15 00		
Citizens of Millville, Cumberland County, ...	110 00		
A Citizen of Somerton, . .	2 00		
Citizens of Salem, ...	35 00		
		1,598 53	
INDIANA.			
From a Sunday School of P. E. Church at Indianapolis, . .		5 00	
MICHIGAN.			
From Congregation of German Evangelical Lutheran Church, Ann Harbor, ...		20 00	
SPECIAL.			
This sum being a premium awarded by Delaware County Agricultural Society at their Fair held at Media, to Messrs. Harveys, Painter, and Barney, for superior Working Oxen, . . .		50 00	
		$27,135 04	18,162 48

to the Fund for the Relief of the Norfolk and Portsmouth Sufferers. Cr.

Amount brought forward, ...		$37,585 01
Expenses continued—		
Amount brought forward, ...	$118 56	
" Cash paid Patrick Ward for attendance on Committee at Board of Trade Room, per voucher 127, ...	5 00	
" Cash paid John Cummings for making out clean copy of Report, and this account current for the Printer, per vucher 128, ...	10 00	
" Cash paid King & Baird for printing, per voucher 129.	3 00	
		136 56
Counterfeit money, ...		35 00
		$37,756 57

Dr. *Thomas Webster, Jr., in Account with the Philadelphia Contributors*

Amount brought forward, .		$18,162 48
Chairman's statement continued—		
Amount brought forward, .	27,135 04	
This sum left with Howard Association, Norfolk, by Dr. A. B. Campbell, the contribution of a Citizen of Philadelphia, . .	50 00	
UNKNOWN.		
This sum handed to Chairman in the street by some person unknown, to be added to some School or Church's contribution, name not recollected, . .	5 00	
IN MERCHANDISE.		
Sundry articles of Merchandise, viz:—Groceries, Tea, Crackers, Wine and Brown Stout, donated to the sufferers, for which the bills were receipted when sent in,	515 50	
This sum in cash received since the public meeting approving the account, ...	15 03	
		27,720 57
		$45,883 05

NOTE.

The following bills for advertising were sent in receipted, and are *not* in the account:

Pennsylvania Inquirer, ...	$160 50
North American, ...	156 82
Morning Times, ...	129 37
Pennsylvanian, ...	158 50
Ledger, ...	30 65
Sun, ...	24 94
Bulletin, ...	82 87
Argus, ...	75 50
Daily News, ...	19 62
Sunday Dispatch, ...	6 00
Commercial List, ...	10 00
Making . . , ...	$854 77

Generously given to the cause, by the proprietors of the above papers.

to the Fund for the Relief of the Norfolk and Portsmouth Sufferers. CR.

	Amount brought forward, . . .		$37,586 01
Nov.	To this sum in hands of Thomas Webster, Jr., Trustee, to pay for Testimonials ordered for Volunteers, and to hand to the Widows and Orphans of the deceased. To Widows and Orphans, .	400 00	
	" Volunteers, ...	1,835 00	
			2,235 00
	To this sum in hands of Thomas Webster, Jr., Trustee, to pay expenses of Printing 5000 copies of Report of Committee, and this account, ...		500 00
	To this sum in hands of Thomas Webster, Jr., Trustee, to pay expenses of re-interment of deceased Volunteers, and to erect a monument to them, . .		2,000 00
	To this sum in hands of Thomas Webster, Jr., Trustee, to purchase Philadelphia 6 per cent. Loans, to be remitted to Orphans' Asylums of Portsmouth and Norfolk, as soon as incorporated, ...		3,000 00
	Balance held as a Contingent Fund, ...		391 58
			$45,883 05

APPENDIX.

Philadelphia, Aug. 15th, 1855.

To the MAYOR of the City of Norfolk:

SIR:—Enclosed please find Drexel & Co.'s (Bankers) draft, No. 1910, at sight, for six hundred dollars, on R. H. Maury & Co., Richmond, Va. This sum is the result of a collection made since 9 o'clock this morning, among a few of the merchants of this city, who have instructed me to remit it to you, to be distributed among the "Howard Associations" of your City, Portsmouth, and Gosport, in the ratio of their respective populations, to aid said Associations in their noble work of alleviating the distress attendant upon the dreadful scourge now prevailing in your midst.

Should there be no Associations of the kind referred to, you will please exercise your own judgment, as the Chief Public officer of the city, regarding its distribution, and hand over to the chief public officer of Portsmouth, and likewise of Gosport, the shares intended for said towns. As the sum remitted is to be divided among the three places, I would suggest that $350 be set apart for Norfolk: $250 for Portsmouth, and $50 for Gosport. You will please acknowledge receipt of same.

A town meeting of our citizens will be held to-morrow, at 12 o'clock M., to adopt a more systematic and public mode of obtaining further relief for your poor.

In haste, respectfully yours,

THOS. WEBSTER, JR.,

No. 7 North Wharves.

Philadelphia, August 16th, 1855.

To the MAYOR of Norfolk:

SIR:—I had this pleasure yesterday, and now inclose you the call for a public meeting, to be held here to-day, at 12 o'clock, M., to concert measures of relief for your city, and its sister towns, in your affliction.

The mail will close at too early an hour to enable the Committee that may be appointed to accomplish anything that could be made available to you to-day.

In all probability, to-morrow's mail will bring you a communication. In the meantime, please send on the address of yourself, and of the Presidents of the "Howard Associations" of Norfolk, Portsmouth, and Gosport, and such other information as may facilitate the Committee in remitting to your Committees; and, until the Committee, or some official of the meeting to be held shall write you—your letter, addressed to me, will find its way to the proper Committee.

Respectfully, THOS. WEBSTER, Jr.

Philadelphia, Aug. 16th, 1855.

Dr. W. H. Freeman:

My Dear Sir:—The meeting to-day dispatched its business rapidly—organized, appointed a Committee, and adjourned. No opportunity presented itself to make known the noble offer of your personal services, and valuable scientific skill towards mitigating the terrible scourge now devastating the seaboard towns of our sister State.

I shall take the chair to-morrow, when the Committee meet, and make known your magnanimous offer. In the meantime, I have funds at your disposal, should you adopt the idea you held forth to-day, and proceed at once by the mail line, at 12¾, noon, to-morrow, for Norfolk.

A letter of introduction to the Mayor of that town is ready for you, and the Committee, which meets at 12 o'clock, M., will doubtless pass officially upon your conduct, and send on to you, and to the public authorities of Norfolk, further testimonials of the high consideration in which they hold your devoted proffer. Very truly, yours, THOS. WEBSTER, Jr.,

Chairman of Committee of Relief.

Philadelphia, Aug. 16th, 1855.

To the Mayor of the City of Norfolk:

My Dear Sir:—Previous communications from me have apprised you that measures are being concerted to dispatch relief to your community, and those of Gosport and Portsmouth. A meeting was held to-day, at 12 o'clock, M., at the Exchange, at which a Committee of fifty persons was appointed to collect funds and remit to you. I have the honor to be its Chairman.

Doctor Wm. H. Freeman, a Philadelphian, and lately a resident of the West Indies, has, with a singleness of purpose, and generous philanthropy that is an honor to human nature, offered his professional services, and visits your city to afford you whatever aid his energy and skill can accomplish.

His credentials and recommendations are of the highest character. The Committee will, at their meeting to-morrow, no doubt act officially upon his magnanimous offer, and send you a copy of the same. In the meantime, I recommend him to your notice.

Very truly, yours, THOS. WEBSTER, Jr., *Chairman.*

Philadelphia, Aug. 17th, 1855.

D. D. FISKE, Esq.,

President of Howard Association, Portsmouth, Va:

DEAR SIR:—Be pleased to find inclosed a draft for four hundred dollars, which dispense, under your Association, to the poor of your town and Gosport.

The Committee of fifty appointed yesterday at the public meeting, will organize at 12 o'clock to-day; and to-morrow I trust to be able to remit you a further sum. The present sum is part of an imperfect collection of a few hours this morning.

Yours, truly, THOS. WEBSTER, Jr., *Chairman.*

Philadelphia, Aug. 17th, 1855.

WM. B. FERGUSON, Esq.,

President of Howard Association, Norfolk:

DEAR SIR:—Please find inclosed E. W. Clark & Co.'s draft, at sight, on John D. Gordon, Norfolk, for six hundred dollars, which apply, through your Association, to the relief of the poor of your city, suffering under the ravages of the terrible pestilence which shrouds your fire-sides.

Yours, truly, THOS. WEBSTER, Jr., *Chairman.*

Philadelphia, Aug. 18th, 1855.

WM. B. FERGUSON, Esq., *Pres't. of Howard Assoc. Norfolk:*

DEAR SIR:—Inclosed please find draft for ($600) six hundred dollars, second remittance on the part of this community to yours, for the relief of the suffering poor of your city, to be dispensed under the superintendence of your Association. Acknowledge receipt. In haste,

THOS. WEBSTER, Jr., *Chairman.*
JOHN TRUCKS, *Treasurer of the Fund.*

Philadelphia, Aug. 18th, 1855.

D. D. FISKE, Esq., *Pres't. Howard Association:*

DEAR SIR:—Inclosed please find draft for four hundred dollars—second remittance on the part of this community to you for the relief of the suffering poor of your city—to be dispensed under the superintendence of your Association.

In haste, yours truly,

THOMAS WEBSTER, Jr., *Chairman.*
JOHN TRUCKS, *Treasurer of the Fund.*

Philadelphia, August 18th, 1855.

D. D. FISKE, ESQ., *Mayor of Gosport and Portsmouth, Va.,*

DEAR SIR:—I had the pleasure this morning when remitting to you $400, and have now, to request you will favour me with correct information of the mortality daily in Portsmouth and Gosport, with such suggestions of what our Committee might send you in the way of relief, that you think proper to add. Are you in want of food and medicines? It is so stated here, and if so, inasmuch as there is no direct conveyance from hence, will funds in cash enable you to procure them?

Do you want doctors and nurses? I have sent three to Norfolk, and the next that offers shall be sent to Portsmouth. Are we right in estimating the ratio of population and suffering as about equal and is 20 per cent. to Norfolk and 40 per cent. to Portsmouth, near the true ratio? The Committee of Relief is anxious to partition all that they may send between Norfolk, Portsmouth and Gosport, in proper shares. Please reply. Yours truly,

THOMAS WEBSTER, Jr., *Chairman.*

Philadelphia, August 18th, 1855.

WM. B. FERGUSON, ESQ.,

DEAR SIR:—By this morning's mail I forwarded to your address a letter containing a bank draft for $600, which I trust was duly received. I also gave two letters of introduction to you—one to W. W. Maul, who is represented as having experience as a nurse in yellow fever, and will volunteer his services to mitigate, as far as his humble efforts may avail, the sufferings existing in your place—one to Dr. Louis Martin y de Castro, a Cuban by birth and a graduate of medicine in this city. Dr. De Castro has seen a good deal of yellow fever in the West Indies, and is familiar with its treatment. He is acquainted with Dr. Freeman, who left here yesterday to give you his services, and will co-operate with him under your disposal. Dr. De Castro brings strong recommendations from two of our Philadelphia Physicians. I would like to have a letter from you, with some suggestions as to what you stand most in need of, doctors, nurses, or funds, and also the relative amount of population and distress between Norfolk and Portsmouth, in order that the Relief Committee here may know how to partition their remittances. I have sent 60 per cent. of collections to Norfolk, and 40 to Portsmouth.

Yours truly, THOS. WEBSTER, Jr., *Chairman.*

By telegraphic dispatch I see the deaths in Portsmouth are

eight per day in a population reduced to 2000. Is this really so? Information about the disease and population and wants of the respective places is very much wanted; as we are all deficient here as to exact data, and the papers are contradictory.

Norfolk, Aug. 17, 1855.

Thomas Webster, Jr., Esq., Philadelphia:

DEAR SIR:—Your favor of the 15th instant, to the Mayor of our city, was handed to us this morning, with its enclosure of check for six hundred dollars, for the relief of the sufferers with the Yellow Fever, and in destitute condition in our city, and in the towns of Portsmouth and Gosport. The distribution shall be made of the amount as requested, with many thanks to the contributors,

I remain your obedient servant,

JAMES A. SAUNDERS,

Secretary, Howard Association, Norfolk.

P. S.—All donations please send to WM. B. FERGUSON, Esq., *President, Howard Association.*

PORTSMOUTH, VA., Aug. 18, 1855.

Thomas Webster, Jr., Esq.

DEAR SIR:—Yours of 17th containing Draft for four hundred dollars, contributions from citizens of your city, for the poor of this community, was received this morning, and the amount shall be faithfully applied as you desire. May heaven reward your fellow-citizens for the aid thus contributed for our suffering people. The fever continues without abatement.

Truly yours, D. D. FISKE, *Mayor.*

PORTSMOUTH, VA., Aug. 20, 1855.

Gentlemen:—I have to acknowledge the receipt of yours of the 18th instant, containing Draft on the Bank of Virginia, at Norfolk, for "four hundred dollars," your second remittance for the relief of the suffering poor in this community. With repeated assurance of respect, and heart-felt gratitude for the liberality of your city,

I remain yours truly, D. D. FISKE, *Mayor.*

THOMAS WEBSTER, Jr., *Chairman*, JOHN TRUCKS, *Treasurer.*

Norfolk, Aug. 20, 1855.

THOMAS WEBSTER, Jr., and JOHN TRUCKS, ESQ.

Gents:—Your valued favor of the 18th inst., enclosing check for six hundred dollars, was duly received, for which please accept the thanks of the Association.

The Fever is still on the increase; some two hundred cases now under treatment. We have lost some of our good citizens, male and female, young and old. Yours, very truly,

JAMES A. SAUNDERS, *Secretary.*

P. S.—Our Association relieved sixty families this morning, in two hours. The distress is very great among the poor. Our office has been crowded all the morning by persons applying for relief, which was granted immediately.

PORTSMOUTH, Aug 21, 1855.

Thomas Webster, Jr., Esq.

DEAR SIR:—Yours of the 20th, containing Draft on the Bank of Virginia, for four hundred dollars, your *third* remittance of a like sum for the relief of our truly distressed community, has just been received. There is yet no abatement of the scourge among us.

May you and your fellow-citizens be abundantly rewarded for the deep interest manifested in our behalf.

In haste, yours, very truly, D. D. FISKE, *Mayor.*

Philadelphia, August 21st, 1855.

WM. B. FERGUSON, ESQ.,

DEAR SIR:—Enclosed please find the fourth remittance from this community to the poor of your city, viz: F. & M. Bank's draft on the Bank of Virginia, for fourteen hundred dollars; receipt of which, please acknowledge.

The Committee are without any favor from you, and inasmuch as your association or no other public body has made any call on Philadelphia, or apprised our community of your sufferings, other than through the papers, the Committee (feel) somewhat embarrassed as to the extent they should proceed in their collections for relief. We are prepared to do all or anything you may suggest; and if you will but intimate what amount of funds you desire to have from this city, it will be sent per return mail. In haste, yours truly,

THOMAS WEBSTER, Jr., *Chairman.*

PORTSMOUTH, Va., Aug. 22, 1855.

THOMAS WEBSTER, Jr., Esq., *Chairman of Relief Committee.*

DEAR SIR:—The illness of our Mayor's family has caused him to refer your communications of 18th, and 22d inst., to me, with the request that I would answer. For him I acknowledge the receipt of the Farmers' and Mechanics' Bank's Draft on the Bank of Virginia, for one thousand dollars transmitted by you, the same being the fourth munificent offering of Philadelphia for the relief of our afflicted and suffering community,

The ratio of population and suffering (40 to 60) given by you for this and our sister city, is believed to be correct, or nearly so. More than half the citizens have fled the town, and the disease is remorselessly seizing upon those who are left, without sparing age, sex, or color. In a present population, of certainly not more than 5000, there are in the opinion of one of our most prominent and reliable Physicians, who is present and has just expressed himself, not less than from three to four hundred cases, and I think his estimate rather under than over the mark. The disease is on the increase, and the daily mortality is now double what it was a week ago. Yesterday there were seventeen deaths ascertained, this morning only up to ten o'clock, there had been ten. No abatement is loooked for before the latter part of next month, and many confidently believe that very few of those who shall remain will escape having it. You will thus perceive that although the mortality is considerable, it is not such as should create the excessive alarm which exists here. But, notwithstanding there are circumstances attending the disease which renders it truly awful, and the bare mention of which will furnish an answer to another interrogatory. I refer to the want of necessary nursing and medical attendance. Four of our most prominent and extensive practitioners have had the disease, and are not able to resume their duties — consequently the few remaining will have more than they can possibly do justice to, although they do all that man may. It is the want of nursing above and beyond all other things, which is felt most severely. Most of those remaining here are persons whose limited means did not admit of flight, and who in health, were rather short of "*helps.*" These poor people, many of them, are sick by families, and very few families are entirely exempt from the prevalence of the idea of contagion. Nurses *cannot* be obtained, friends desert, and in very many cases there is not a soul to attend the sick and dying, but the undertakers, employees, (his hearse driver, and driver's companion, both colored men,) to put the dead into their coffins and graves. Literally the sick attend the sick, and almost literally, "the dead bury their dead." It is this craven fear and inhuman desertion in the hours of illness and suffering, which casts a reproach upon our people, and makes some shudder with horror. I know of no medicines needed but Quinine. There are about 30 ounces in Portsmouth, which is but a small supply. If a quantity could be forwarded by Adams & Co.'s Express, it would place us under great additional obligations. We are not in immediate want of provisions, and to answer another of your interrogatories, without, by any means intending to solicit further pecuniary aid from your "*city of brotherly love*," I think money can be used with more advantage than provisions. In conclusion, sir, I will be frank with you. *Our population is mainly a mechanical one, and most of our people are dependent on daily labor for support.* This disease has deranged every department of business, and is prevailing to a greater or less degree in almost every family. The result is, great, and general destitution prevails. Returning my thanks and those of the whole community, I remain yours, very truly, JAS. G. HOLLADAY, *Member of Council.*

P. S.—I am free to confess that I had answered your letters without perusing them. It is only since I had concluded the above reply, that I read yours of the 22d. I would say that Portsmouth has made no call on any quarter for aid. She has made known her distress, and her sister towns and cities have voluntarily come forward to her aid. To none of them is she more indebted than to Philadelphia. We have received your voluntary contributions, and you now come forward voluntarily and call on us to make known the amount of our wants, and you will furnish the necessary relief by return mail. It is impossible for me to ascertain the extent of our necessities. All the information in our possession has been furnished in foregoing statements. But for your city's part, kindness, and her magnificent humanity shadowed forth in her request to know the extent of our calamity, and determination to relieve it, she has the heart-felt gratitude of a grateful people.

Norfolk, Aug. 22, 1855.

THOMAS WEBSTER, Jr., ESQ., *Chairman.*

DEAR SIR:—Your several favors of 18th and 20th are at hand. We acknowledge the receipt of the six hundred dollars enclosed in yours of the 18th and 20th instant, and now acknowledge the receipt of six hundred dollars enclosed in yours of the 20th.

Mr. Maul has arrived and is at work. Dr. De Castro has also arrived and is doing good service.

In regard to your other inquiries, as to what we stand in need of, we can scarcely say. *Good nurses* we want; we can get a good number of persons to help, but they are not *nurses.* We have in the city at least 280 patients under treatment with the Fever. Our Doctors, so far, hold out nobly. Our friends in Portsmouth, in this respect, are not so well off, as they wrote yesterday to Baltimore for medical aid.

As to the population, it is in favor of Norfolk two to one, generally, but both are so decimated by "run-aways," that it is impossible to judge how they stand now, but we think that at least two-thirds of the people of Norfolk have left — and suppose Portsmouth at least bears the same proportion.

As to the deaths in Portsmouth, I am sorry to say that there is some truth in it — will ask them to send you, if possible, a daily report. In our city yesterday, we had fourteen deaths; to-day up to this time (12 o'clock) eleven deaths. The Fever has now assumed a form that it attacks all classes, old and young, black and white.

Should your kind letters not be promptly and satisfactorily answered, do not think hard of it, as we have so much to do and so few to do it.

In regard to our thanks for your kindness, what shall we say? Words are useless; but every one of our hearts are full of thankfulness and gratitude for our Philadelphia friends.

In much haste, D. WHEELER, *Secretary.*

Portsmouth, Va., Aug. 23, 1855.

THOMAS WEBSTER, Jr. *Chairman of Relief Committee.*

DEAR SIR:—Yours of the 22d, containing a Draft for four hundred dollars, the fifth remittance from you for the relief of the sick and destitute of our town, has been received, and, be assured, sir, that the hearts of many have been made to rejoice, even in their afflictions, by the extreme liberality of your city.

Dr. Rizer and Mr. Graham arrived to-day, and their services will be most cheerfully accepted.

With grateful feelings for your efforts in behalf of the suffering here, I remain, yours truly, D. D. FISKE, *Mayor.*

Norfolk, Aug. 23, 1855.

THOMAS WEBSTER, Jr., Esq., *Philadelphia.*

DEAR SIR:—Your highly esteemed favor of the 21st, enclosing a check for fourteen hundred dollars, was duly received, but not in time to reply by return mail, which closes in an hour after the mail from the north arrives.

The Fever is still on the increase, and we see no chance of its abating. The weather is very unfavorable. We have over three hundred cases now under treatment in the city, and seventy or eighty cases in the Hospital. If you have any Physicians accustomed to the practice of Yellow Fever, also nurses, please send them to us. Dr. Higgins, one of our best Physicians, was taken with the Fever last night. He had eighty cases before this. By his illness it increases the duties of our Physicians, who are much fatigued. The deaths from 2 o'clock yesterday to 12 to-day, are fifteen. Baltimore supplies us with provisions. You will oblige us by continuing your remittances, as the requirement of aid from this office is very great. Yours, very truly,

JAMES A. SAUNDERS, *Secretary*.

Norfolk, Aug. 23, 1856.

THOMAS WEBSTER, Jr. Esq., *Chairman of the Relief Committee, Philadelphia.*

DEAR SIR:—Your favor of the 22d instant, with check enclosed for six hundred dollars, came duly to hand; the receipt of all your kind donations have been acknowledged. Our mails are very irregular; we are almost cut off from even mail facilities; our city is nearly depopulated.

The disease has commenced its ravages upon the colored population, and there are many of them down with it. The Fever is still increasing, and the weather is very unfavorable. It is really distressing to listen to the appeals at this office for relief. Nurses and Physicians we want; we have but few of the former, and are all employed.

Unless we have cool weather for some eight or ten days, we must expect a large increase of the Fever. Our Hospital is nearly full, and we are making arrangements to accommodate double the number. We fear that the disease will be as bad in September, as at this present time.

Doctors Freeman and De Castro are doing good service; they are attending the sick day and night, and doing all the good that lays in the power of man. The nurses sent by you are untiring in their efforts, always at their duty as men. We have sent Mr. Spriggman to Portsmouth, where they are destitute of nurses, and have also sent three Physicians to that city, who arrived here to-day from Baltimore, there being only three of the Faculty remaining to attend to the whole town. The Fever is still on the increase in Portsmouth and Gosport. I will keep this open till to-morrow at 12 o'clock.

Yours, very respectfully,

JAMES A. SAUNDERS, *Secretary*.

Portsmouth, Aug. 25, 1855.

THOMAS WEBSTER, Jr., Esq., *Philadelphia.*

DEAR SIR:—Your favor of the 24th, with the draft for eight hundred dollars, the sixth remittance from you, has just been received. I have only time to acknowledge its arrival, having three sick in my own family to nurse, besides other numerous pressing duties to attend to.

Several Doctors and nurses, recommended and sent by you to our relief, have arrived and entered upon their labors of love.

May God bless them and you, is the prayer of
Your obedient servant, D. D. FISKE, *Mayor.*

Philadelphia, Sunday, August 26th, 1855.

D. D. FISKE, ESQ., *Mayor of Portsmouth.*

DEAR SIR:—I avail myself of the quiet of the day to review our correspondence, and to make a few suggestions which the bustle of the morning (mail closing at ten o'clock) would prevent. In order that my fiduciary accounts may be correctly audited, I ask your attention to the annexed statement of monies remitted to you, which please examine and if the same is found to be correct, advise me accordingly, that it may be for me, a voucher to our Committee, up to this period.

August 15th.	To the Mayor of Norfolk, to be handed to you, (being an individual effort at collecting before a public meeting was called,)	$ 250
17th,	to yourself, Clarke & Co.'s dr'ft on Gordon,	400
18th,	" Far's & Mec's B'k d'ft on B'k of Vir.,	400
20th,	" " " " "	400
21st,	" " " " "	1000
22d,	" Clarke & Co's draft on Gordon,	400
24th,	" F. & M.'s B'k d'ft on B'k Va., at Rich'd,	800
25th,	" " " " "	400
	Total,	4050

independent of Medicines. I sent by the Mail Agent yesterday one hundred ounces of *pure Quinine*, marked "Howard Association, Norfolk," with instructions to supply you; it should have been received by you *this* morning. I now enclose you an invoice of medicines for your association, which I have had put up, and which, with 15 boxes of lemons, went by Adam's Express to Baltimore yesterday, freight free, and should be at Portsmouth by Tuesday morning, at the very latest. The list is no doubt imperfect, as there was not time to ask professional advice upon it; but the articles are from an old and reliable house, and can be warranted. If there is any drug, medicine, chemical, restorative, or tonic, or article of diet, which you are out of, or which you think you will want, or that your doctors can suggest, let us know by telegraph or mail, and it shall be sent immediately. Quinine is manufactured here probably better than anywhere else in the United States, *it* and calomel are so often adulterated that it has occurred to the writer that it would be but proper for you to have your whole supply direct from the laboratory, and then you would be sure of having it *pure* and of *uniform* potency. What say you? There are rare preparations of iron, of French manufactures, iodines, &c., &c., to be had in this city from the importer; but as the undersigned is no doctor, he can't say if they would be useful in yellow fever. Your doctors can reflect on it. Should you not have liberal quantities of Bay Rum, Cologne Water, aromatic vinegar, and such washes, and likewise abundance of lemons, arrow root, tapioca, sago, bare barley and oatmeal for the convalescent, let us know. I telegraphed to know if you wanted an apothecary, to put up the prescriptions. By the sea steamer of Wednesday, if not before, I will send supplies assorted as we best can. The steamer will meet some of your boats in the Roads, and trans-ship the supplies.

In conversation with my friend Professor Chas. D. Meigs, of the Jefferson Medical College, this afternoon, he suggested that you apply at once to Government for tents, and that you remove the healthy part of the population from the town to an open elevated region, taking good care that the encampment shall be dry, airy, and full of comforts. It is not requisite to go far, a half a mile or so would answer. Sometimes the boundary and limit of infection is well defined, and *beyond it* all is healthy, no matter how proximate. *To remove out of the infected district is the surest of all plans to avert the pestilence*, in his opinion. I give you the substance of his remarks, as well as I can remember them. I shall try, to-morrow, to send you by the mail train, in the care of the Mail Agent, some pure Ice Cream, from Delaware County, Pa. I have asked Physicians here about it, and they tell me the sick and the convalescent could not have a better article. It is of peculiar excellence in this vicinity, and if I can make the arrangements, you shall have a daily supply for the sick. I hope to send you more money, doctors and nurses to-morrow. Yours truly,

THOMAS WEBSTER, Jr., *Chairman.*

A Letter of the same tenor sent to the Howard Association, Norfolk.

Philadelphia, August 27th, 1855.

D. D. FISKE, ESQ., *Mayor of Portsmouth, Va.*,

DEAR SIR:—Herewith enclosed please find Farmers' and Mechanics' Bank's draft on the Bank of Richmond, for nine hundred and nine 17-100 dollars, the eighth remittance from this community to yours in their distress. This contribution is made up of one day's pay of the master workmen, mechanics, and laborers employed at the navy-yard in this city, and same amount has been sent on. It is not the intention of this Committee to publish the names of any contributors to the fund, but this is an exception to the rule. Very many of these generous hearted men have worked in your town and Gosport, and have had, and expect to have again, social relations with your people. It has been a great pleasure to the Committee to transmit you funds, and I trust it will not be deemed insidious to any, to say that there is a gratification about this remittance surpassing any other. The true dignity of labor could have no better exemplar than the genial and free handed sympathy our mechanics and laborers offer to your "*Mechanical town.*"

Yours truly, THOMAS WEBSTER, Jr., *Chairman.*

Philadelphia, August 27th, 1855.

HON. WM. L. MARCY, *Sec'y of State, Washington.*

SIR:—A Mr. D. W. Baynon, formerly of Pernambuco, informs me that he, in connexion with others, through Mr. Consul Lilly, about a year since, made a communication, in writing, to your department, of the mode of treating yellow fever at Pernambuco and that it is on file. I have to request that you order a copy to be sent to D. D. Fiske, Mayor of Portsmouth, Va., and one to Wm. B. Ferguson, President of the Howard Association, Norfolk, Va., with information that it is by request of this Committee. And further, I have to ask the favor of a copy for this committee. It being the cause of humanity itself that is believed to be at stake, you will pardon me if I urge that *promptness* and punctuality be given to this request.

Yours truly, THOMAS WEBSTER, Jr., *Chairman.*

Philadelphia, August 27th, 1855.

WM. B FERGUSON, ESQ.,

DEAR SIR:—D. W. Baynon, of Pernambuco, calls to say that about one year ago a full and detailed account of all the facts connected with the yellow fever at Pernambuco, its origin, manifestation, mortality, and the most successful treatment of it, was sent on by Mr. Consul Lilly of that port to the

Secretary of State. I immediately wrote to Mr. Marcy, requesting him to send a copy of the same from the files of the department to D. D. Fiske, Mayor of Portsmouth, and Wm. B. Ferguson, President of the Howard Association, Norfolk, Va., and a like copy to this Committee. Mr. Baynon further states that as near as he can recollect, the treatment was to give an emetic immediately upon the first manifestation of the disease, followed by the mildest cathartic, the patient to be supplied freely with pulverized ice—ice itself, not ice and water. External application of mustard to the feet, abdomen, and calves of the legs. Hot mustard baths, as hot as can be borne by the patient, to the extremities, and ice on the head, in extreme cases, and extreme cases only—that he has seen the black vomit itself cured by *pulverized ice* itself, given freely internally.

I have only time to hand you the enclosed, and to say that I have sent you two apothecaries, a doctor, and three nurses today, August 28th. Yours truly,

THOMAS WEBSTER, Jr., *Chairman.*

DEPARTMENT OF STATE,
Washington, Aug. 28, 1855.

THOMAS WEBSTER, Jr., Esq., *Chairman of the Committee for the Relief of Norfolk sufferers, Philadelphia.*

SIR:—I have received your letter of the 27th instant, requesting three copies of a Report made in April, 1854, by Mr. William Lilley, United States Consul, at Pernambuco, on the mode of treating Yellow Fever at that place.

You are informed in reply, that in the latter part of the year 1853, a communication was received at this Department, from the Sanitary Commission, of New Orleans, "instituted for the purpose of investigating the origin, modes and limits of extension, and general character of the epidemic of that year," requesting that a number of circulars prepared by the Committee, might be forwarded, through the medium of this Department, to certain Consuls of the United States, residing in places, occasionally or periodically visited by the Yellow Fever. In these circulars were embodied many questions respecting the meteorology of the "locality" on which the Report was to be made; also, in reference to its soil, water, and drainage, its position in regard to rivers, marshes, &c., the character and social condition of the population, number of cases and deaths among the different classes, character of the epidemic, its symptoms, progress, duration, and termination, and its propagation by exposure to an infected atmosphere, personal communication with the sick, and contact with goods or clothing.

The Reports of the Consuls were sent as they were received to the New Orleans Sanitary Commission, whose elaborate Report, embodying the results of the labors of the Sanitary Commission, has been published by authority of the City Council of New Orleans.

I take pleasure in transmitting to you one of the *two* copies now remaining in the Department, containing Mr. Lilley's Report. I am, respectfully your obedient servant,

W. L. MARCY.

Portsmouth, Aug. 29, 1855.

THOMAS WEBSTER, Jr., Esq., *Philadelphia.*

DEAR SIR:—We have again to acknowledge the receipt of a check, in yours of the 27th instant, for nine hundred and nine dollars and seventeen cents. You have been most kind indeed, and in the name of the Mayor and the people of Portsmouth, I offer you our heart-felt thanks for the munificent manner in which aid has poured into our laps from your fraternal city.

Our Mayor is down with the prevailing epidemic, I saw him this morning, and shook his hot hand.

Very truly, yours, H. WILSON,
Treasurer of the Fund for the Relief of Portsmouth.

Philadelphia, August 31st, 1855.

D. D. FISKE, ESQ., *Mayor of Portsmouth.*

DEAR SIR:—Mr. Peete's letter is just to hand. I have nothing in cash to send you, and am in debt a few hundred dollars; but by Monday I trust to be able to remit you more. We have lost, by the Railroad accident, one of our best co-laborers, G. W. Ridgway, Esq., crushed to death in an instant; he leaves a wife and little ones.

I have given an introduction to Mrs. Olive Whittier, a widow, aged fifty-five, who insists upon going, and refused one to a Miss Patterson, aged eighteen, (a recent convert to the Roman Catholic faith,) who insisted upon going. I positively refused; but may yet have to give her a letter. The five "Sisters of Mercy" have not yet left. I have written to know why. Miss Patterson is not a Sister, but was to have gone with them. If you can send back the Ice Cream cans and tubs, I need not pay for them. Mineral Water bottles should be preserved, if possible, as they are paid for. Deem it not parsimonious to call your attention to these items, for their value can be realized by your community in cash through the Committee.

I hope soon to hear of your recovery. Why don't you remove your healthy population, and starve the fever? Old Point, the Rip Raps, or any hill-top, invites you. Pardon the freedom of my remarks, but after all, *removal from infection* is the surest plan of subjugating the fever.

Yours truly, THOMAS WEBSTER, Jr., *Chairman.*

Saturday afternoon, Sept. 1st.

Fathers SHERIDAN, McNANNY, & McGOVERN,

REV'D SIRS:—A Miss Leonora Patterson, aged eighteen, a recent convert to your Church, persists in offering her services to go to Portsmouth as a nurse in yellow fever. She has been advised by me not to go. She claims the *right* to go. because she intends devoting her life to religion and charity. Will you have the kindness to let me know something relating to her? I have thought you might be cognizant of her state of health, or of some information which would induce you to remonstrate with her against going. I believe it is because Miss M. M. McCredy, Miss O'Neil, Miss Josephine Carroll, and others, "Sisters of Mercy," are going there, that Miss Patterson desires to go. I am yours truly,

THOMAS WEBSTER, Jr., *Chairman.*

Philadelphia, Sept. 1st 1855.

D. D. FISKE, ESQ., *Mayor of Portsmouth, Va.*,

DEAR SIR:—In the discharge of my duty as Chairman of the Committee of Relief, I have been perplexed to know how to pronounce upon an application made by a Miss Leonora Patterson, aged eighteen, to go as nurse to your assistance. Miss Patterson is a recent convert to the Roman Catholic Church, and intends devoting her life to religion and charity; therefore, viewed in connexion with that resolution, her determined and persistent application for a letter of introduction is not surprising. I have written to the three pastors of her church for their opinion. I have remonstrated with her, but she says she will go, because, for one reason, among the Sisters who are going are some of her friends, and further, that she feels she ought to go. I have deferred giving her a letter till your expected letter arrives, 5 P. M., under the hope that you will say positively that you are not in want of any more nurses; promising her if your advices are different however, or if there shall be no letter at all, to give her an introduction to you. Were I a Catholic, possibly I could see this sacrifice in another light; as it is, I have to decide, and for the soul of me I cannot resist her earnest solicitations to go. I have deferred yielding to her request, put her off till to-day, and begged her to remain; but she will go, if not from this Committee, by her own agency and means. So my dear Sir, take her by the hand and let her go to the chambers of the sick, and fill the sphere to which she devotes herself. Watch over her too, for though she may prove a comfort and help to you, still she may, and I fear will want relief from you herself.

THOMAS WEBSTER, Jr., *Chairman*

Philadelphia, Sept. 1st, 1855.

REV. JOHN MCGOVERN, *St. Paul's Church.*

DEAR SIR:—I addressed a note to you this afternoon relative to the application of Miss Leonora Patterson to go as nurse to the poor of Portsmouth, Va., now suffering under the ravages of yellow fever. I have written a letter of introduction for Miss Patterson, and from her conversation, I recognize you as her guardian, and therefore place the letter (enclosed) in your hands; two passes and a five dollar note, for incidental expenses. It is for you, my dear sir, to say whether she ought to go, or not. I leave the case in your hands.

Very respectfully,

THOMAS WEBSTER, Jr.,

Philadelphia, Sept. 5th, 1855.

WM. B. FERGUSON, ESQ.,

DEAR SIR:—Please find enclosed Farmers' and Mechanics' draft on the Bank of Virginia, at Richmond, Va., for $403, being the tenth remittance from this community to yours in its distress.

I have nothing to reply to from your association—no advices since Mr. Wheeler's letter of the 28th, and consequently, no acknowledgment of Remittances on the 28th and 29th ult. Our Committee met yesterday, and to the queries of What is the condition of things at Norfolk? What can we do for them? and many of like tenor, I would only reply by reference to Mr. Wheeler's letter of the 28th, and the newspapers. If our efforts to assist you are not up to your expectations, do not blame us; we want information, and you will confer a favour to this community if you will see that we have a daily report from Norfolk. We get it from Portsmouth. Yours truly,

THOMAS WEBSTER, Jr., *Chairman.*

Philadelphia, Sept. 5th, 1855.

MR. THOS. WEBSTER, JR.,

I called at your office yesterday, for the purpose of ascertaining whether with your assistance I could introduce at Norfolk a remedy and positive preventive of yellow fever. I was directed to call upon you by Mr. Everett, No. 4 North 9th street. If you take any interest in this, you can get any information you wish of him. I expect that any profit arising from the introduction of it to be mutual. Yours,

JOHN STREET, No. 588 North 10th Street.

Philadelphia, Sept. 6th, 1855.

JOHN STREET,

SIR:—Enclosed I return you your letter of the 5th. "*Profit*" in the distress of Norfolk and Portsmouth is not within the province of this Committee's business, and empiricism is not to be thought of for a moment.

THOMAS WEBSTER, Jr., *Chairman.*

Philadelphia, Sept. 6th, 1855.

WM. B. FERGUSON, ESQ.,

DEAR SIR:—Enclosed please find Girard Bank's draft for three hundred dollars, being the eleventh remittance from this community to yours. I have still to say that I have no advices from your association later than the 28th ult. Yesterday I sent you Chloride of Zinc, one barrel and one puncheon of Lime Juice. To-day I am sending you a barrel spunges, fifty dozen Mineral Water, Chloride of Zinc, and six dozen of Aromatic Vinegar. I would send you Ice Cream or anything else you might want, if you would but advise us. A Mr. Robert Harvey has desired me to send for two orphan children, viz: Cassells and Eugene Harvey. Enclosed is the statement, with directions where to find them, and likewise a ten dollar bill, to defray the expenses of sending them on; if they can be sent on free, apply the ten dollars to your wants—it is part of our fund. I enclose my private card, that the children may know where to come upon arrival here. Waiting your letter, I am,

Yours truly, THOMAS WEBSTER, Jr., *Chairman.*

Portsmouth, Sept. 5, 1855.

THOMAS WEBSTER, Jr. Esq., *Philadelphia.*

DEAR SIR:—Learning this morning that Dr. Martin Rizer, who has been very much indisposed for several days, anticipates leaving to-day for your city — I take great pleas-

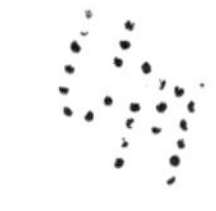

ure in tendering him a letter to you. Dr. Rizer's exertions have been most arduous and unremitting—it would have been impossible for any one to have exerted himself more energetically. His services have been most efficient and successful, and he has won the confidence of our citizens to an eminent degree, consequently he will leave greatly regretted.

I tender you, sir, my acknowledgements for the obligations you have placed me under in sending a gentleman so deserving.

With profound respect, I am, dear sir, your ob't serv't,

JAMES G. HOLLADAY.

Philadelphia, Sept. 11, 1855.

WM. B. FURGUSON, Esq.,

President of Howard Association, Norfolk.

Care of S. S. STUBBS, Esq.

DEAR SIR:—I address this letter to the care of your Ex-Mayor, because I have had nothing from your Association since the 28th ultimo, and with the hope that I may learn that this, as well as my previous respects covering remittances have been received. The mail closes at 11 o'clock A. M. By the courtesy of the Post Office Clerks, I have been able to get letters addressed to you covering remittances, bills of lading, &c., in the mail *after* the hour of closing, (an unusual thing,) and for this special reason, as well as others as a business man, I should like acknowledgments of receipts of the remittances sent to you.

I am aware how death has thinned the ranks of your Association, and how impaired your clerical force has become; still, it would take but a moment to write "Yours of —— with —— enclosed, is received; send us more."

Herewith enclosed is Farmers' and Mechanics' Bank's draft for $3000, the fourteenth remittance from our community to yours, receipt of which please acknowledge. Your orphan children are objects of special sympathy here, and you will greatly oblige us by stating the number of them, and imparting as much information to us relative to them as you can. It is with rejoicing that we learn you are moving your population away from the infection.

The Episcopal Churches, by recommendation of Bishop Potter, took up collections on Sunday last; and it is owing to that in a great degree, that the Committee are able to remit the enclosed sum. Yours truly,

THOMAS WEBSTER, Jr., *Ch'm.*

Philadelphia, Sept. 11, 1855.

S. S. Stubbs, Esq., Norfolk:

Dear Sir:—To *insure* an acknowledgment of receipt of a remittance sent this day to President of Howard Association, (from whom we have had nothing since 28th ult.,) I herewith enclose the letter containing same, to you.

Yours truly, THOMAS WEBSTER, Jr., *Ch'm.*

Philadelphia, Sept. 11, 1855.

Wm. B. Ferguson, Esq., Norfolk:

Dear Sir—My letter of to-day, to you, covering $3000, is sent enclosed to address of S. S. Stubbs, Esq.,

Yours truly, THOS. WEBSTER, Jr., *Ch'm.*

Philadelphia, Sept. 11th, 1855.

Thomas Webster, Jr., Esq.,

Dear Sir:—In accordance with the request you made of me at 8 o'clock on Saturday morning last, I left here in the one o'clock train of the same day, and arrived in Norfolk about noon on Sunday. I presented your letter to Mr. Ferguson, President of the Howard Association, who said, when he had read it, that he was both glad and sorry to see me—glad, because it showed that Philadelphia kept up her interest in Norfolk, and sorry, becarse I would certainly have the fever, and he had not the nurses to attend to me. I told him I had had the fever eight years ago. In reply, he said that he would not then take the responsibility of ordering me to leave without a consultation of the most eminent physicians now in Norfolk, but that Dr. Marsh, of Philadelphia, who had for some years resided in the South, and had there, some years ago, had the yellow fever, was now down with it, and had quite a severe attack. That his was by no means the only such instance, and that every physician from the North was either dead or sick. That they really had not the nurses to attend them, and that there were now in Norfolk more than enough of physicians from the South to attend upon the sick.

Accordingly, in the afternoon I was waited upon by four physicians from New Orleans, Augusta and Norfolk; after a conversation with me they retired, and in the evening Mr. Ferguson handed to me a letter, of which I enclose to you a copy. Yesterday morning Judge Olin, of Augusta, Georgia, the present Secretary of the Howard Association, gave me the enclosed letter to you.

Nothing therefore remained for me, but to return to Philadelphia, which I have done.

By the kindness of some of the physicians there, I was enabled to see about three hundred cases of yellow fever, and to make two post-mortem examinations, during the 24 hours I remained there. I have the honor to be, very respectfully, your obedient servant, A. B. CAMPBELL.

Norfolk, Sept. 9, 1855.

DR. A. B. CAMPBELL.

DEAR SIR:—Fully appreciating your kind and valuable tender of services as a physician to our heart-stricken community, I feel it my duty, after consultation with our acclimated physicians, to decline your kind offer, *they* believing that your noble offer would only be attended, after a short practice of usefulness, with, perhaps, a sacrifice of your life.

Again I thank you, and through you to Mr. Webster a heart-felt appreciation of his and your kind attention.

Respectfully, W. B. FERGUSON.

P. S.—I have requested the Doctor to particularly request Mr. Webster not to send any more unacclimated physicians or nurses. Between man and man they are adding only fuel to the flame. Things look better.

Norfolk, Sept. 10, 1855.

THOMAS WEBSTER, Jr., Esq., *Philadelphia.*

DEAR SIR:—Whilst fully appreciating the motives that have influenced you in sending to our plague-stricken city, a gentleman of such decided character and medical experience as Dr. Campbell, we are constrained by a stern sense of duty, to decline accepting the tender of the Dr.'s services at this time. The sad experience of the past few weeks has proved to us most conclusively that every northern man who comes amongst us, is doomed to fall a victim, adding to the already heavy burden of grief under which we labor. Besides this, the illness of so many physicians took off the services of nurses and attendants from the sick of our city, and we feel impelled by a sense of honor and sympathy, to have those cared for who come among us at the risk of their lives in obedience to the high dictates of humanity. This last, however, would be a trifling consideration were it not coupled with the loss of valuable lives. We have a large number of southern acclimated physicians now in our midst, and others are coming to the rescue, so that the sick will not suffer from want of medical attendance. In taking the step which duty has pointed out to me, we must be understood as intending no disrespect to Dr. Campbell; on the contrary, we feel extremely grateful to him, and justly estimate the noble instincts that have prompted his visit, Respectfully, yours,

W. MITE OLIN, *Secretary.*

Philadelphia, Sept. 12th, 1855.

WM. B. FERGUSON, ESQ.,

DEAR SIR:—Our Committee met yesterday, and to the solicitude expressed for the welfare of your community, I could only reply as at the meeting previous—"There is nothing from the Howard Association since the 28th of August," and refer them to the newspapers.

Last evening, however, Dr. A. B. Campbell called at my dwelling, and handed me a letter dated 18th inst., from your Secretary, W. Mite Olin, informing us that you had sufficient medical aid, and that you had declined Dr. A. B. Campbell's proffer of professional services.

Dr. McCay, of Georgia, who assisted the faculty at Savannah, last year, and whose services you have also declined, has called this morning, and tells me likewise that you have now a full force of physicians.

I am rejoiced to hear your medical corps is so well organized.

Permit me to remark, however, that this Committee, while anxious to serve your community as much as lies in its power, and in such a way *only* as may be agreeable to your Association, think in Dr. Campbell you would have found most efficient aid. He is a practitioner of the highest character, great nerve and endurance, and has had large experience in yellow fever and malignant diseases generally, at the U. S. Military Hospital at Vera Cruz, and as Chief Resident Physician of our extensive Almshouse.

I shall be happy to hear from you, and to furnish you with anything you may desire. Only let us know your wants, and they will be relieved as far as lies in our power. Yours truly,

THOMAS WEBSTER, Jr., *Chairman.*

Extract from the Baltimore *American:*

"I regret to announce to you that Dr. De Castro was compelled to leave yesterday for his home in Cuba, and that Drs. Freeman, of Philadelphia, and Peniston, of New Orleans, will also leave either to-day or to-morrow. All these gentlemen have done noble service in the cause of humanity since they have been among us, and their names will be almost held sacred by the survivors of this pestilence. I have seen a great deal of them, and in reference to them I speak "that I do know." Other doctors have, doubtless, done as well, but I have not been thrown with them as I have with those I have mentioned, and therefore cannot speak knowingly of them.

"Dr. Freeman I can never forget. No reward that man could give would be a sufficient compensation for his noble conduct. He was in attendance upon little Mary Eliza Starke, to whom he showed a devotion equal to that of a mother for her first born. The child, as she drew near her end, seemed inspired by the good angel that hovered over her to carry her spirit to the God who gave it. She spoke as never child spoke before. Her thoughts were altogether of heaven, and Dr. F., was fully capable of sympathising with and responding to them. She named a hymn which she wished him to sing to her—he sang it. She named a prayer she wished him to pray for her—he prayed it. He read to her from the Holy Bible, he unfolded to her the true piety of his noble heart, and both as physician to her body and mind, performed his duty most skilfully, most faithfully. God bless him! But, alas! the Almighty fiat had gone forth. The beautiful child followed her father through the death region; her mother commenced her eternal journey last night, her aunt and little sisters will, in all probability have commenced theirs, ere I write you again. Great God! Thus are whole families swept off by the fell destroyer, leaving not a trace behind.

Philadelphia, Sept. 15th, 1855.

Wm. B. Ferguson, Esq.,

President Howard Association, Norfolk, Va.

Dear Sir:—Enclosed please find Farmers' and Mechanics' Bank's draft on Bank of Virginia, at Richmond, for nineteen hundred and twenty-six dollars and fifteen cents, being the fifteenth remittance from this community to yours, in its distress, and making the total amount from us to you, up to this date, in cash, independent of all other contributions, fourteen thousand dollars, ($14,000,) receipt of which please acknowledge.

I am pressed with many offers from persons who represent themselves to be acclimated to fever climate, and who have had, and nursed in, Yellow Fever in various places; some that have nursed in other fevers in French Military Hospitals, on shipboard in putrid fever, in Water Cure establishments, &c. But, of course, I refuse introductions, since I have heard from you that you do not want more aid. This is not enough to deter some who, under the idea that their skill as nurses *must* be of service, have gone on to offer their services to you, upon their own account, and with their own means.

Returned nurse, Nathan Thompson, is going around the adjacent country, buying live chickens, and will start to-morrow for Norfolk, with about 200 pair. Returned nurse, W. W. Maull, will go back to you to-morrow. Returned nurse, Wm. Driver, will go back to you at once, if wanted.

I have written communications from chemists, suggestions of all kinds from various sources, about the purification of your city, sent to me in writing. Offers of gifts of chlorides, and other disinfectants, &c., &c., and can, if you desire it, engage a corps of resolute, acclimated men, (at least said to be,) who will go down and act as scavengers, white-washers, and work at cleansing and purifying under your control and authority. I am sending you Ice Cream to-day. I have engaged some barrels of toasted bread; will send it to-morrow, with directions for use. If you can attend to enclosed request without dispensing with more urgent business, please do so. The Harvey children have not come yet.

Yours truly,
THOMAS WEBSTER, Jr., *Ch'm.*

A Letter of same tenor sent to Portsmouth.

Philadelphia, Sept. 18th, 1855.

JAMES G. HOLLADAY, Esq., Portsmouth:

MY DEAR SIR:—Your esteemed favor of the 16th is at hand. Our call for volunteers was responded to by men who have been, and are, an honor to our community. Some have fallen, martyrs, and not to *their* surprise. They knew the risk, and when I put it strongly before them, as was my duty, the cool, calm courage of their replies, showed them to be actuated by the highest feelings of human nature. Poor Mercer—you know, perhaps, his history— * * * He gave as his reason for going to your assistance, that "he could nurse well, and that it was the duty of man to assist his fellow man in times of pestilence;" and he has *now* rendered up *his* life to the cause of humanity. Barrett was, indeed, a noble fellow; and, had he lived, his intelligence and lofty views of his profession would have insured a life of great beauty and usefulness. I shall call on you, after a little, for a return of the length of service, and order of merit, of all the doctors, nurses, and druggists sent to you, in order that this Committee may have proper data to base their estimation of them. It is our intention to get up handsome gold medals for the survivors, and to inter the dead, and erect a suitable monument over them. In haste, yours truly,

THOMAS WEBSTER, Jr., *Ch'm.*

Portsmouth, Sept. 10, 1855.

THOMAS WEBSTER, Jr., Esq., *Philadelphia.*

MY DEAR SIR:—Your favors of the 6th, 7th, and 8th, have been handed me; that of the 7th covering check for two hundred dollars, and that of the 8th, a check for five hundred and two dollars and fifty cents. The 6th calls my attention particularly to the inquiry and solicitude of Bishop Potter, which I have just answered in a letter to him. I have seen his sister, and all are doing well at present. In relation to the articles you mention, the letters will be handed to those having charge of such matters.

And now, my dear sir, how am I to find language to express my thanks to your community, for the untiring zeal which it has so constantly and enduringly manifested towards our distressed and suffering people? There are feelings and sentiments, the character of which cannot be described by language, because they are of too spiritual a character. Such are the emotions of gratitude which now agitate me. When these trying times are over, if I shall be alive, I will take the liberty and exercise the delightful privilege of making known to our people, publicly, the estimation in which your benevolence is held, your continued and often repeated kindness, and the zeal and more than fraternal willingness which you have manifested towards us. These, when I contemplate for a moment, fill me with gratitude, and act as the rod of old, causing the apparently hard rock to gush forth, in evidences of hidden, but living fountains. * * * * I am, truly and sincerely, your ob't serv't,

HOLT WILSON, *Treasurer.*

Portsmouth, Sept. 13, 1855.

THOMAS WEBSTER, Jr. Esq., Chairman.

MY DEAR SIR:—I have your favors of the 10th and 11th, together with one from Solomon Shepherd, Secretary. We feel deeply obliged to the Rev. Mr. Spackman, for his unselfish offer to come on here, and, as it were, enter the jaws of death which are open to receive almost every stranger that comes in our midst. We cannot consent to such a sacrifice—even if we thought his services among our destitute people were well nigh essential to their well being, here and hereafter.

Express to him the profound respect we entertain for his noble and more than generous offering up of himself in the holy cause in which he is engaged. We thank him most gratefully, but must decline his services.

And now, my dear and kind sir, send us no more of your generous people. We will not consent to the sacrifice of the lives of such men. If it must be so, and we are to die without medical aid, which we require to be acclimated, why let us die — but spare your own self-sacrificing and generous men. You have been — and still continue to do so — pouring into our afflicted borders the grateful contributions of a generous and noble brotherhood. This is enough. Let this suffice — but spare your people. Such men may be required among yourselves in some future day of affliction; but which, I pray God may forever avert.

I acknowledge the receipt of a check for two thousand dollars. I pray you to thank in language which fails me, the various brotherhoods and individuals in your more than brotherly city towards us, for their munificent gifts, and for their ennobling and enlarged sympathies.

Yours, most truly, HOLT WILSON, *Treasurer.*

Norfolk, Sept. 13, 1855.

THOMAS WEBSTER, Jr., Esq.,

MY DEAR SIR:—I am in receipt of yours of the 11th, enclosing letters to the President of the Howard Association, of Norfolk, which I have handed to him in person. He desires me to acknowledge the receipt of your draft for three thousand dollars; and to express to you, and through you to the benevolent and humane of your city, the grateful thanks of this suffering people, for this, another renewal of their kindness.

He desires me to acknowlege the receipt of one can of Ice Cream, two boxes of wine, and one box of clothing. He also desires me to inform you, that the Association have upon its hands two hundred and seventy orphan children, which have been specially provided for. The Lecture Room of Christ Church, a neat and comfortable building, in a pleasant part of the city, has been, for the present, appropriated to their use. Kind and good nurses have been provided and every attention paid to them.

W. W. Maul, about whom inquiry is made, has had the fever, but is up, and has gone to Baltimore for a few days, and expects to return. Mrs. Ann M. Caust has not had the fever, she is doing good service, and at her post. The deaths from old cases yesterday equaled in number that of past days —some 40; but the number of new cases fell short of that of previous days. Number of interments in Elm Wood and Cedar Grove Cemeteries, from fever, up to to-day, (13th September,) are eight hundred and ninety-two; in the Catholic Burying Ground, one hundred and twenty; in the Jews' Burying Ground, (supposed to be) twelve; at Julappi Hospital, about two miles from the city, thirty; at Old Hospital, (containing the dead from Barry's Row, where the fever first broke out) forty; making in all, one thousand and ninety-four.

The above statement has been furnished to the President of the Howard Association, but falls short, I think, cf the number of whites that have been interred. In addition to the interments at the places above named, many who died where they had friends, were taken to the cemetery, and many that left the place after the disease commenced, have died abroad. Moreover, this does not embrace our colored population, slave and free, among whom the mortality has been awful. I doubt not the loss of our people, all told, has been, up to this time, more than two thousand.

With grateful acknowledgments, I am truly your friend and obedient servant, SIMON S. STUBBS.

P. S.—The President begs leave to inform you, that the pressure of unceasing labor, and the smallness of their force, has caused him to neglect that punctuality which ought, and otherwise would, have been paid to their very kind friends abroad. S. S. S.

Portsmouth, Sept. 16, 1855.

MY DEAR MR. WEBSTER:—I have but this moment declined the services of Mr. Etasse, who presented himself with a letter of introduction from you, and high testimonials from others who seem to have had every opportunity of judging him. The manner of the tender was such, evincing so determined and disinterested desire to render aid to the suffering, that I was reluctant to refuse his request to be put on duty for fear of wounding his feelings, while on the other hand, from the respect inspired, I was but the more disinclined to accede to his wishes, and thereby devote him to destruction. For our experience here within the last six or seven days admonishes us that none may come from the North and hope for impunity. This gives me occasion to refer to some of your people who now sleep beneath our soil, and of whom I should have written you to-day. I refer to Singleton Mercer, Edmund Barrett, and Miss Johnson.

Each of the above named individuals served us with zeal and fidelity, and their deportment throughout commanded my highest commendation. Mercer, you knew well by reputation, doubtless, and it is needless for me to say anything of him. But of Barrett, who may have been a stranger to you, I cannot forbear particular mention. On his first arrival he was employed as a nurse, but was soon placed in a drug store to compound prescriptions. While acting in the capacity of nurse, his intelligence, gentlemanly manners, and kind deportment so won upon all with whom he was thrown in contact, that the demands upon his exertions were unremitting, and after being wearied out by his labors as apothecary, during the day, he would yield to solicitations, (against my advice) and sit up with the sick again all night. * * * * * *

In this way I am cut off for time, and have either to give Mr. Etasse no letter at all, or this unfinished one. Believe me, my dear sir, that I, in common with all our people, entertain for your community, no ordinary emotions of regard. You have no idea of the embarrassments the few of us labor under, and must pardon much. Two hours ago I was compelled to stop writing, and it has been utterly impossible to resume, and even now, I am surrounded by an unusual crowd.

Respectfully, yours, JAMES G. HOLLADAY.

Norfolk, Sept. 17, 1855.

Thomas Webster, Jr. Esq., *Philadelphia.*

Dear Sir:—Your esteemed favor of the 14th instant, is at hand, enclosing a draft on the Bank of Virginia, at Richmond, for nineteen hundred dollars, being kindly contributed by the citizens of Philadelphia for the aid of the sufferers here, which amount will be faithfully applied to aforesaid purpose. Please accept our most sincere thanks.

Very truly, yours, R. W. BRODIE, *Treasurer.*

Portsmouth, Sept. 17, 1855.

Thomas Webster, Jr., Esq., *Philadelphia.*

Dear Sir:—Your esteemed favor of the 14th and 15th, I have before me—the former remitting a check for eleven hundred and twenty-nine dollars and sixty-five cents, being the sixteenth remittance from Philadelphia to this community in its distress, making the total of remittances from your benevolent Committee, in cash, independent of all contributions of medicines &c., the mnnificent charity of ten thousand dollars. Generous Philadelphia, may the charitable echoes from your renowned metropolis resound throughout the land, proclaiming your noble deeds, which should be known of all men, as a brilliant example, and one most worthy the imitation of all. Our gratitude is unfeigned, and our thanks are heart-felt. You do well to refuse all applications from the noble men who wish to aid us by their personal services. We cannot, under the circumstances, consent to accept their services. The generous offer to cleanse and purify our streets and town, by the noble band of resolute men whom you mention, and who are ready, with your scientific chemists, to come on and do the work, I feel bound also to decline, with sincere thanks for their unbounded kindness. We have received lime, chloride, and other disinfectants, from Baltimore, which we hope to use beneficially, and which we hope will, in some measure, supply the offer you have been so forward to make. Well nigh all the articles, the Ice Cream, the Toasted Bread, the Oranges, the Lemons, have been received, and are refreshing and nourishing to the weary and the feeble.

There is a pleasant and refreshing breeze from the North this morning, though the sun is hot and disagreeable. The Physicians say the disease is abating. There are fewer new cases, and these have assumed, it is said, a milder type. It is most devoutly to be wished that this may be, and will continue so.

Yesterday the Rev. James Chisholm, who has spent himself in his parochial duties, and in ministering to the spiritual need of all who asked for his services, was buried. His memory will be frought with melancholy interest to our people, when they learn his self-sacrificing devotion to the duties of his vocation. Meek and unpretending, he was yet firm and unswerving where duty pointed. He was attacked while reading the burial service at the grave of a child, and expired in a few days after, at the Naval Hospital. I am truly happy to apprize you that Dr. Bryant, of your city, is well, has left the Hospital and is in town. Dr. Hamill is also convalescent. I saw Dr. Rizer this morning; he is again sick with the fever. His devotion to us, and the cause of human suffering, brought him here originally, and he is here again to prove his steadfastness. I trust he will not be very sick; he seems to be doing well this morning, and I fondly hope will be suffered to pass through unharmed. I have, my dear sir, written you a long letter, and fully. You are entitled to every consideration by us, especially to full and grateful responses.

I am, very truly, your ob't serv't, HOLT WILSON.

Philadelphia, Sept. 27th, 1855.

"*Howard Association, Norfolk:*"

I drew from bank, funds for your Association, under the full impression that I should certainly hear from you by the mail of yesterday; and upon not hearing, I am constrained, from a sense of my duty to all interested, to put it back in bank. I am aware your President is deceased. Who his successor is—whom to address—what your wants—are all left to conjecture. And I therefore must earnestly request you to communicate with me. Captain Thompson went down on Monday with stores, and goes down again on Saturday with a fresh supply. Yours truly,

THOMAS WEBSTER, Jr., *Ch'm.*

Philadelphia, Sept. 28th, 1855.

President of Howard Association of Norfolk.

DEAR SIR:—I herewith enclose you an invoice of merchandise bought for your community, by Captain Nathan Thompson and myself, receipt of which please acknowledge.

On Monday next, we shall forward from here about two hundred pairs of live chickens, and about 300 pounds fresh butter. All that we have sent you in the way of medicines, provisions, &c., has been at our own instance, and not at your request or suggestion. As soon as we heard of a want, we endeavored to relieve it. For some of the stores we have had acknowledgments of receipt, but not for much the greater part. Being left to our own conjectures and inferences is not near as satisfactory to our Committee as the daily receipt of orders and suggestions would be, and upon the completion of the present engagements for chickens and butter, we shall rest and wait your suggestions and requisitions. It will afford us great pleasure to execute an order immediately upon its receipt.

Of the clothing sent you for the children, there are thirty-five suits of woolen, made by the tailor of the Girard College for the Orphans living under the care of that institution—and sold to us at the same price as to the Girard College—the cloth, cut, and make, being identical in quality and style.—Your little fellows need feel no pain in wearing apparel the same as the boys of the most munificently endowed college in America. Our children's contribution is kept intact, to be applied, when completed, to the *permanent* relief of your orphan children only. About this I wrote to the late Mr. F., on the 2d, asking if he had any suggestions to make.

With the hope that I may be able to have a copy,

I am, yours truly, THOMAS WEBSTER, Jr., *Ch'm.*

Extract from Letter of Mayor of Norfolk, dated Sept. 27th to Volunteer Physicians.

The annals of our civilization furnish no authentic record of a visitation of disease as awfully severe as that which we have just encountered. Out of an average population of some 6000 souls (much the larger portion of whom were negroes—a class less liable than the whites to the fever in its more fatal forms,) about 2000 have fallen—a proportion of nearly *one* to *three*—and but few have escaped an attack of the disease. We are now a community of convalescents.

Had we not received *material* aid from abroad—had not the different portions of our country sent their heroic delegations of physicians, nurses, and stalwart co-laborers—had not noble spirits volunteered to the rescue, (to die, if need be, like Curtius for Rome,) our people must have *sunk* beneath the burden of their agony. There was a period, about the first of September, when the evil seemed greater than we could bear.—Corpses lay unburied—the sick unvisited—the dying unattended. Our surviving physicians were either sickening or becoming exhausted; our remaining population was panic-struck at the sight of accumulating horrors and duties. You, who visited us for our relief, were astounded at the unrealized state of things which you found here—an evil the like of which you had never before witnessed. But, nerving yourselves to the task, and telegraphing for reserves, you went resolutely forward with your science and its accompaniments, carrying aid where it was most needed, and infusing vigor into many hearts that would otherwise soon have ceased their painful throbbings.

Your noble bands, too, have experienced a worse than decimation, though many of you were acclimated to the disease in other latitudes before coming hither. A list, which has been carefully prepared from the original entries, and handed to me by Franklin H. Clack, Esq., of New Orleans, (our efficient temporary Chief of Police,) shows that, out of eighty-seven physicians and assistants who visited us during the space of thirty-three days previous to the 19th instant, *twenty physicians are numbered with the dead!* This is exclusive of the mortality among our resident physicians, *more than half of those abiding here having died!* No better evidence of the pure self-devotion of the martyr-like spirit, which has actuated your Samaritan associations in hastening to our relief, can be furnished.

Sept. 28th, 1855.

THOMAS WEBSTER, Jr., Esq.

MY DEAR SIR:—Your favor of the 27th is at hand. The death of our former and lamented President prevented the correspondence being attended to as it ought; in addition, our Secretary has been ill, so that I am appointed Corresponding Secretary, and I promise in future all letters shall be answered. I would have replied to yours by return mail, but it is so arranged that we do not get our northern letters until about the time the mail closes, which renders it impossible for us to reply. Every thing seems to operate against us, except the kind liberality of friends, which seems to know no bounds. This is particularly the case in regard to your city. I am instructed by the officers of the association to request you to send no more articles of provisions, unless ordered by an officer of this association. But whatever you have to contribute, let it be in money, or its equivalent, if possible. I am glad to say the fever is rapidly abating. Very few new cases, and only three deaths to-day. Many of the poor people are left entirely destitute, and will have to be supported entirely by the charitable for a long time. The kindness of your people will be kept in grateful remembrance by us. Truly yours,

SOLOMON CHERRY, *Cor. Sec.*

Norfolk, Oct. 1, 1855.

THOMAS WEBSTER, Jr., Esq., *North Wharves.*

MY DEAR SIR:—Your esteemed favor of the 28th, per the hands of Mr. S. S. Stubbs, was handed to me this morning. You have, doubtless, received mine before now making some explanation for seeming negligence on our part.

The articles, I think, have all been received, of which your communication advises us. Please, my dear sir, accept our sincere thanks for your unremitting kindness in our behalf, and at the same time let me assure you that, in future, all of your communications shall have attention. You have, doubtless, seen in your papers, the proceedings of a meeting of our Association, appointing new officers &c. Let me again request you in future to make us a remittance in funds, of whatever your kind and generous people may bestow.

I am, truly yours, SOLOMON CHERRY, *Cor. Sec'y.*

Norfolk, Oct. 5, 1855.

THOMAS WEBSTER, Jr., Esq., *Philadelphia.*

MY DEAR SIR:—I have none of your esteemed favors unanswered. I take pleasure in acknowledging the receipt of the chickens and butter by this morning's boat. Please accept our thanks, not only for these, but for your kind and unremitting attention to us throughout the whole of our affliction.

I regret to say Dr. W. H. Freeman, of your city, leaves us to-day. This distinguished gentleman has taken our people captive. By his gentlemanly deportment, his untiring energy, and his unsurpassed skill, he has won all hearts. He seems to us a near and dear friend, and it is with much regret we have to give him up. Philadelphia may be proud of such a son.

Yours truly, SOLOMON CHERRY, *Cor. Sec.*

Portsmouth, Oct. 8th, 1855.

THOMAS WEBSTER, Jr., Esq., *Philadelphia.*

DEAR SIR:—Mr. Holladay has just handed me your letter of the 4th, he is still feeble, and unable to reply to it. He highly appreciates your kind sympathy, and desires me to say as much. In a few days he will be out again.

The disease has nearly burnt out. There is no material in town for it to feed upon. Nine-tenths at least of the white population have passed through, and I believe that thirty-five per cent. of them have died. The blacks, for the first thirty days of the epidemic, did not seem to be liable to take it. After that time, the cases among them became very frequent until probably two-thirds were attacked. But there was a marked difference in the mortality of the two races, the ratio of deaths among the Negroes being only from five to eight per cent. The mulattoes suffered more in proportion than the blacks, but not so much as the whites. The period of illness among our colored population rarely extended beyond three days, and there was very little treatment necessary.

Our principal wants are for staple articles of food and clothing. The time for luxuries and dietetics has passed. We have very few sick people, and the convalescents are gradually going to their accustomed employments.

Capt. Johnson is still employed. He has been most faithful and attentive. It is probable that he will remain with us as he has employment at the Navy Yard offered him. Mercer as long as he lived, acted his part well; so did Barrett and Graham. Very respectfully, your ob't serv't,

J. H. SCHOOLFIELD, *Ch. San. Com.*

Portsmouth, Oct. 11, 1855.

THOMAS WEBSTER, Jr., Esq., *Philadelphia.*

DEAR SIR:—It is with much pleasure, through the goodness of an all wise Providence, that I am able to acknow ledge the receipt of your kind favor of the 9th inst., covering a list of doctors and nurses from your city who have been on duty here, and to whom you gave letters of introduction to me. In consequence of the severe and protracted illness with which I was visited, I had the satisfaction of becoming acquainted only with a few of those named in the list, and could not, from personal knowledge, fill the blanks as you desired. I have, however, referred the matter to Dr. Schoolfield, the Chairman of the Sanitary Committee, who will attend to your request as early as possible. By the way, you may see the Doctor in a day or two, as he informed me he should visit your city during the present week.

I trust that at a future time, some suitable expression may be made, on behalf of our poor and afflicted people, of the gratification that pervades every heart for the deep-felt sympathy and unparalleled liberality manifested by the citizens of Philadelphia, and many other places. Language, adequate to an expression of my own feelings in reference to the cordial expressions of sympathy, the large sums of money, and the bountiful supplies of provisions, &c., which have been poured in upon us, and without which our sufferings must have been an hundred fold, is not at my command.

With grateful feelings and prayers for the health, happiness and continued usefulness of each member of your Committee,

I remain, sir, yours truly, D. D. FISKE, *Mayor.*

Philadelphia, Oct. 26th, 1855.

THOMAS WEBSTER, Jr.,

DEAR SIR:—Do me the favor to present to the Committee my very sincere thanks for the honor they have done me, both by selecting me as one worthy to represent the Medical profession of Philadelphia at Norfolk, and by offering for my acceptance so valuable a testimonial. Tell them that when you called upon me to request me to go, you offered me compensation, and that I declined all remuneration whatever, preferring rather to bear my own charges.

I went because your Committee requested me to go, and did but my duty, without the hope of fee or reward. I therefore with a grateful heart decline their costly gift, preferring, if it so please them, that the amount designed for the purpose, may be given to the widows of those physicians from Philadelphia, who died there. I have the honor to be, very sincerely,

Your friend and servant, A. B. CAMPBELL.

Portsmouth, Oct. 23, 1855.

THOMAS WEBSTER, Jr., Esq., *Philadelphia.*

DEAR SIR:—I have your esteemed favor of the 18th, but it came to me too late to reply by return mail.

I am afraid that Dr. Schoolfield spoke almost too positively in reference to the founding of an Asylum. It is very true, this subject has presented itself to the minds of our Committee, and has been alluded to among ourselves individually, and I am aware that such an appropriation of a surplus fund is regarded as a legitimate one. But such cannot be agreed upon and settled as a fixity yet, not knowing the amount of our indebtedness, and not being in a condition to ascertain that amount at present. As to our having $30,000, that I could not aver. But we certainly shall have a surplus of some thousands. A large portion of such I should be pleased to see set apart as a charity fund, if I may so call it, to be expended, or rather returned to the prolific sources of generosity whence it emanated—when pestilence or other calamity may in the future be caused to visit our kind and distant friends.

The Doctor was right, however, in advising you not to remit any further funds at present, for, if we have ample means to defray the expenses incurred, we ought, perhaps, to return what may be remitted for this purpose, or appropriate it to our Orphan Fund.

I am quite sure that the graves of the Philadelphians can be identified—they were all marked. Dr. Peete informs me that there were forty-eight orphans. How many more there may be who may be required to be cared for, we cannot say.

Frederick Muhsfeldt died, as I learn from Dr. Peete, and a youth in the drug establishment where Barrett was engaged. No number of the Transcript contains all the names of the victims—and the copies containing the daily mortality are exhausted. Mayor Fiske designs hereafter publishing them in one issue, which he will be pleased to forward to you when it appears. Yours, truly, HOLT WILSON.

Philadelphia, Oct. 30th, 1855.

HOLT WILSON, Esq.:

DEAR SIR:—Your esteemed favor of 22d, was duly received. Our Committee have instructed me to close up my account, and we will remit remainder of fund for use of orphans. Give me the names of the Trustees of your Institution, that I may purchase stock, and have it transferred to them in trust, for those made "orphans by the pestilence," and also the number of orphans.

I have read your letter with great interest, and agree with you in your views of the surplus funds that you have in hand. So far as regards our contributions, we do not expect you to return anything. We have sent the contributions to a committee in whom our community, and yours, too, have deservedly great confidence; and *their* disposition of any surplus, will no doubt be guided by the same philanthropic motives which has prompted the contributions from all parts of the Union. Our remaining fund, as I have said, will be specially remitted.

I am engrossing the account for publication, and should like to add thereto a concise narrative of the fever, and would like you to furnish me with your history of it. Can you not write it out for me, taking care to note the date of first case, progress, mortality, population—positive and comparative—ratio of mortality, medical force resident at the time, loss of life among them, number of volunteer or non-resident physicians, mortality among them, &c., &c. Let it be authentic.

We shall print five thousand copies of account current and report. Yours, truly,

THOMAS WEBSTER, Jr., *Ch'm.*

Portsmouth, Va., Nov. 13th, 1855.

THOMAS WEBSTER, JR., Esq.,

DEAR SIR:—Since my last letter to you, two facts in relation to the origin of yellow fever at this place, have come to my mind, which, I think, have an important bearing. Towards the latter part of July, after the Ben Franklin had been sent from Portsmouth, two lighter-men, Noah Wickers, a mulatto, and George Trotter, a negro, were passing the steamer, having a load of wood for sale. They were hailed from the Ben Franklin, and went along side. The wood was purchased of them, and delivered by them. This was on Tuesday. A gale of wind sprung up, which prevented them returning home, and they were compelled to remain and sleep on board the steamer. They left on Wednesday, and reached home the next day, at Brown's Hill, eight miles from Portsmouth. Both of them sickened on the day they arrived at home, Thursday, and died, with well-marked symptoms of yellow fever, on the seventh day afterwards.

Jones, Chief Engineer of the Ben Franklin, joined her after she reached our port. He went on board while she lay at Gosport, about the 27th June, sickened with the fever on the 3d of July, and died at the Marine Hospital, where he was sent, on the 6th. Respectfully, your ob't servant,

J. H. SCHOOLFIELD.

Portsmouth, Nov. 26, 1855.

THOMAS WEBSTER, Jr., *Chairman of Relief Committee.*

MY DEAR SIR:—I am at last able to forward you a list of the orphans, in accordance with the request you made in a previous favor. The list is yet imperfect and there are many more to be added. The Rev. Thomas Hume furnished me with the inquiry, from which I forward you the enclosed copy.

Yours, truly, HOLT WILSON.

Philadelphia, Nov. 26th, 1855.

TAZEWELL TAYLOR, Esq., Norfolk:

DEAR SIR:—The Committee of Relief for Norfolk and Portsmouth sufferers, in this city, in closing up their accounts, will have a surplus of $3000, one half of which is for the orphans of your city, and the other half for the orphans of Portsmouth. I am instructed to purchase Philadelphia six per cent. loans, and to convey same to the contemplated Orphan Asylum, which the Howard Association say will be organized, so soon as said Institution is duly incorporated, and I am furnished with the proof of the fact, its corporate title, &c. Meantime the investment will be made. Our council here advises the Committee to have legal advice upon the subject in Virginia, as "trusts often fail for want of speciality." My object in writing to you is, to request you to draw a deed of trust, by which Thomas Webster, Jr., Chairman for the citizens of Philadelphia, donates ——— (Philadelphia six per cent. Loans)——— to ——— (Orphan Asylum, of Norfolk, in trust,) ——— for the maintenance and education of Orphans, according to the rules of said Asylum. The revenue only, is to be expended for the purpose. I have apprised Solomon Cherry, Esq., Corresponding Secretary of Howard Association, that I have written to you on the subject. I presume the Howard will have no objection to our application to you for your professional advice as to the form of a deed, and that you will cheerfully furnish us with the same. Yours, truly,

THOMAS WEBSTER, Jr., *Ch'm.*

Norfolk, Nov. 29, 1855.

THOMAS WEBSTER, Jr., Esq., Philadelphia.

DEAR SIR:—Your favor of the 29th instant is received, and I regret that pressing duties have prevented my earlier attention to it. It will afford me pleasure at all times to aid you and your generous fellow-citizens in carrying out your noble and benevolent purposes in behalf of the orphans of our city, and for which myself and my fellow-citizens will be ever grateful.

I learn that an act of incorporation will soon be obtained for an asylum, and when this is procured, no difficulty can arise as to secure the appropriation of the fund in any manner you may wish. And until the incorporation is had, there can be no donation to it and no necessity to make any deed of trust which could only be made, until there be some individuals in trust to assign it to the corporation when created, and this would in effect be but to change or substitute some other person than yourself as trustee for a brief space.

All that will be necessary hereafter will be to transfer the 6 per cent. to the corporation in trust to have the interest (for &c.,) as you may choose to limit it.

I venture this suggestion for your consideration with the assurance that you may command my services in any way, should you still require them in this matter.

I am, very respectfully, yours,

TAZEWELL TAYLOR.

Philadelphia, Dec. 15th, 1855.

SOLOMON CHERRY, Esq.,

DEAR SIR:—I have sent our account current and report to the printer, and would like to add, in the appendix, a statement of the whole number of cases in Norfolk, and the whole number of deaths, so that it would show the extent of the pestilence. Can you not send me such statement per return mail?

Yours truly, THOS. WEBSTER, Jr., *Ch'm.*

Portsmouth, Dec., 18, 1855.

THOMAS WEBSTER, Jr., Esq., *Chairman of Relief Committee.*

DEAR SIR:—Your letter to Mr. Holladay, owing to his absence in Court, did not reach him until last night. Being still engaged he has requested me to reply to it.

Annexed, I give you a table, as near correct as circumstances will permit me to make it.

	Population during fever.	
Whites,	2,200	
Blacks,	1,800	
		4,000
Cases, Whites,	2,100	
" Blacks,	1,700	
		3,800
Deaths, Whites,	890	
" Blacks,	95	
Whites per cent.,	$42\frac{1}{3}$	
Blacks,	$5\frac{1}{4}$	

This estimate, though made in round numbers, is very little from the truth. The number of deaths is nearly absolutely accurate, as I have been diligently engaged in preparing it for publication for the last two months. All agree in saying, that there were not two hundred persons who escaped an attack, of all that remained in town.

The first cases occurred on the 30th of June, in a house on Allen & Page's ship yard, where the Ben Franklin was undergoing repairs. It began to decline after the 20th of September, and disappeared, with the exception of a few standing cases, by the 10th of October. There were two cases among the returned refugees after the first of November.

Very respectfully, your ob't serv't,

J. H. SCHOOLFIELD, *Ch. San. Com.*

Norfolk, Dec. 18, 1855.

THOMAS WEBSTER, Jr., Esq., *Chairman of the Relief Committee.*

DEAR SIR:—I am in receipt of your esteemed favor of the 15th, this morning, and hasten to reply. I regret that it is out of my power to give you the desired information. We have no data by which we can give anything like a correct number of cases, nor can we even give the number of deaths with that certainty which is desirable. A. B. Cooke, Esq., our President, has been engaged for the last few days in making up a list of the dead, and he requests me to say that 2,100 is about as accurate as he can make it. Owing to the great consternation, confusion, &c., about the time the fever was at its worst, no correct account was kept. We have the register kept by the keeper of our cemeteries, and we find 600 burials whose names are unknown. I regret that it is out of my power to furnish you with the information sought. I am engaged in making up one for publication, and will furnish you with copies of it when published.

Our Association has been incorporated by our Legislature, now in session. It was the first act of the Assembly. As soon as we can have it printed in pamphlet form, I will forward you a copy of that also.

Yours, truly, SOLOMON CHERRY.

Norfolk, Jan. 1st, 1855.

THOMAS WEBSTER, Jr., Esq., *Philadelphia.*

DEAR SIR:—I am in receipt of your esteemed favor of the 31st ult., and hasten a reply. I am much obliged for your kindness in forwarding the copy of our Act of Incorporation to

Mr. Hunt. In fact, we owe your city a debt of gratitude which we can never cancel, for your many and continual acts of kindness.

I have been engaged in making up the account of our Association. It is a very perplexing and almost interminable one. When completed and published, I will send you copies of it.

It is with much regret, in reply to your queries, that I have to be the communicator of melancholy tidings. Such has been my painful duty in many instances, however recently, and now I have to add another to the list. James Hennessy arrived in this city on or about the 9th of Sept. He was taken to the City Hospital (or rather the "Howard Infirmary"), on the 15th, and died on the 17th. Thus, in this instance, you will see how malignant was the epidemic.

Is it the intention of your Committee to have the remainder of the doctors and nurses who died here, removed to Philadelphia? If so, when? My object in making this inquiry, is this: Our Association has purchased in the "Elmwood Cemetery," four lots. In one, we intend to place the remains of all the doctors who volunteered their services and died here; in another, the remains of the nurses; in another, we will bury the orphans who may die under our charge, and the remaining lot is intended for the Members of the Howard Association. Thus, in close proximity, will meet the remains of those who struggled together during the fearful epidemic that so ravaged our city.

If it would be agreeable to your people, it would be gratifying to ours, if you would allow the remains of your lamented volunteers this resting place. It seems to me to be a very appropriate one. Do not understand me at all, as attempting to dictate; but merely to express a desire that would be agreeable to our members. The city of Charleston has sent on a fund to erect tombstones over the remains of those of her sons who fell here. We shall, so soon as it is prudent, remove them to this spot, where the monument will be erected. I am truly, yours,

SOLOMON CHERRY, *Cor. Sec.*

Philadelphia, Jan. 2d, 1856.

SOLOMON CHERRY, Esq., *Sec'y. Howard Association:*

DEAR SIR:—Your favor of yesterday, in reply to my respects of 31st ultimo, is just received. I have communicated to Mrs. Hennessy the painful news of the death of her husband in September last. Her suspense has doubtless prepared her for this information.

It has been resolved in our Committee, in obedience to the wishes of the families of deceased volunteers, to bring on their remains to be re-interred here, and to erect a suitable marble monument to their memory. This will be done. I shall see you, personally, during the winter, about this matter.

Your intention regarding them is proper, but the wishes of the wives, mothers, and sisters of the deceased, ought to guide both your Association and our Committee. Yours truly,

THOS. WEBSTER, Jr., *Ch'm.*

P. S.—Our report is in press, and ought to be out during this week.

Portsmouth, Jan. 4, 1856.

THOMAS WEBSTER, Jr., Esq., *Philadelphia.*

DEAR SIR:—In reply to your questions about the asylum for orphans, I have to say that there has been some little delay in the house of delegates in relation to the act incorporating it. Mr. Holladay will go to Richmond to-morrow, and as soon as we get a bill through I will inform you. Very truly, yours, HOLT WILSON.

NAVY YARD,
Monday, Sept. 17th, 1855.

DEAR SIR:—I send you the following memoranda for *your* information:

Received in Naval Hospital, from August 1st to Sept. 14th, citizens of Portsmouth, men, women, and children,		405
Discharged, cured,	213	
Died,	138	
Remaining,	54	
		405
Persons attached to Navy,		91
Cured,	37	
Died,	28	
Remaining,	26	
		91

All fever patients.

Very respectfully,

E. F. OLMSTEAD, U. S. N.

DR. WM. H. FREEMAN,
National Hotel, Norfolk, Va.

Report of Howard Infirmary, Norfolk, from opening to closing.

Number of white patients admitted up to 5th October,		188
Grown up, male,	99	
Grown up, female,	33	
Children, male,	34	
Children, female,	22	
		188
Number of deaths up to 5th,		100
Grown up, male,	67	
Grown up, female,	23	
Children, male,	6	
Children, female,	4	
	100	
Number disch'd up to 5th,		77
Grown up, male,	40	
Grown up, female,	15	
Children, male,	12	
Children, female,	10	
	77	
Sent to Orphan Asylum,		11
		188

Mortality among white, 51·34 per ct.

Colored Ward.

Number admitted,		84
Discharged,	77	
Deaths,	7	
		84

Rate of mortality, 8 per cent.

*REPORT.

Report of the Joint Committee of Councils relative to the malignant or pestilential diseases of the Summer and Autumn of 1820, in the city of Philadelphia.

To the Select and Common Councils of the city of Philadelphia.

The Joint Committee appointed to "*inquire into the facts connected with the appearance and prevalence of malignant or pestilential disease, during the past Summer and Autumn, and to report those means they may deem best adapted to prevent its recurrence, or to check its progress,*" beg leave to report,—

That the best expedient for obtaining the information contemplated by the Resolution of Councils, appeared to be that of a public invitation to Medical Societies and individuals; and the following one accordingly issued from several newspapers, viz:

"The Select aud Common Councils, at their last meeting, appointed a Committee to inquire into the facts connected with the appearance and prevalence of malignant or pestilential disease, during the past Summer and present Autumn, and to report those means they may deem best adapted to prevent its recurrence or to check its progress. That Committee respectfully invites the College of Physicians, the Academy of Medicine, the Board of Health, the Lazaretto Physician, the Port Physician, and others, to communicate answers to the following questions, viz:

First. Had you an opportunity of observing any cases of malignant fever in Philadelphia, in the months of July, August, September, and October, 1820?

Second. In those districts which, according to your experience, were most affected by disease, what peculiar causes were discovered, which did not exist in other parts of the City?

Third. Did the disease abate in any considerable degree before the appearance of frost.

Fourth. What means should be adapted with a view of preventing the recurrence, or of checking the progress of malignant autumnal fever, in this City?"

The design of your Committee, in limiting their queries to those above written, was to produce information that might be relied on as the foundation of an improved police, without eliciting those points of discrep-

---

* This report having been pronounced by high authority to be one of the most important in its recommendations of police and sanitary regulations as a means of preventing yellow fever that has ever been published, it has been deemed advisable to insert it.

After two months diligent search, a copy of it was ascertained to be in the possession of John McAllister, Esq., who has politely loaned it to the Committee for republication.

ance in scientific discussions which have frequently arranged the medical faculty into parties.

The College of Physicians were the first to send their answer, which is annexed, marked A.

The Academy of Medicine communicated the paper annexed, marked B.

The Port Physician conceived that his sentiments were sufficiently expressed as one of the Committee of the Academy of Medicine.

The Lazaretto Physician sent the paper marked C, hereto annexed.

Dr. Currie sent the paper annexed, marked D, and Dr. Emlen the paper annexed, marked E.

It will be perceived that those Societies and the Lazaretto Physician have formed their opinions and advice on the strength of facts which they have not offered in detail, and that for these they refer to the Board of Health.

The statement of this Board, then, thus recommended, cannot fail to receive the greatest attention. This is annexed, with the publication it refers to, and is marked F.

One of the chief objects of your Committee was to obtain statements of facts; and another, to have the benefit of opinions founded on them. It is well known that the learned Societies who first acceeded to the invitation, have hertofore differed in their sentiments respecting the origin of malignant fevers with which the cities of the United States have been afflicted; but your Committee are now happy to observe an unusual degree of coincidence as regards the cause, and entire consent respecting the means of prevention. This unity of the Medical parties consists in their belief that the city *may become unhealthy, even to the malign state, from offensive matters brought in vessels from other ports*, and that *a deleterious atmosphere may arise among us, from accumulated filth about the wharves and streets, from the want of cleanliness in families, and from inadequate ventilation.* It is not essential for the purpose of effective legislation, that the City Councils should seek for nice distinctions in Physiological points, or that they should inquire, without a prospect of attainment, into the degree of concentration of miasm necessary to produce or disseminate febrile diseases. Is is enough for them to know that the *Summer pestilence* of our cities, if not exactly the same, is no less terrific in character and termination than are intertropical diseases; and that physicians of all parties agree in the important opinion, that neither of them *will be likely to spread in a pure atmosphere.* If then the disease in question originate in filth, here or abroad, in a cellar, a street, or a ship; or if, being generated by whatever cause, in whatever place, *it has the power of propagation only in foul air*, your Committee would recommend the immediate adoption of measures calculated to prevent its regeneration from domestic, as well as its retroduction from foreign sources; such, too, as will probably check its progress, if those precautions should prove unavailing. The Medical faculty of our city has recommended the revision and strict observance of the health laws, and more assiduous attention to cleanliness. Your Committee had commenced an inquiry with a view to the emendation of the former, when they were assured that the Board of Health, assisted by eminent physicians, were employed in the work. To that board the subject more properly belongs, and your Committee have declined interference. It is understood that the contemplated revision will embrace the sections of the law relating to Quarantine, as well as to domestic nuisances; and especially the power of enforcing the former, and removing the latter. If the Councils should find themselves called upon to act, your Committee respectfully intimate that the fit period for interposition will be after the publication of the projected alterations of the laws, or when it shall be ascertained that no progress towards the improvement of these will be made.

The existing powers of the Board of Health, and of the City Councils, are limited to the express or implied terms of their respective charters. All their powers could not be specifically defined; but the usage of either of those bodies has been such as to confer the legislative portion of municipal regulation on the Councils, while the Board performed the duty of enforcing such of the ordinances of the former as related to health. The Councils enjoin their own officers to execute the ordinances, and the Board of Health, though independent of the Corporation, have been accustomed to lend their aid.

Many nuisances may arise in Summer, not to be prevented by contemplation of law; the Board of Health therefore intend to apply to the State Legislature for additional powers, to enable them, *as cases arise*, not only to judge what are public nuisances, but to proceed promptly to the suppression of them. As, for example, where a person is attacked by any malignant disease that may probably extend, it would be proper that the Board should have direct powers to remove any local annoyance from houses or vessels that may have occasioned it, and that the neighbours should be sent away at their own or public expense, lest they contract the malady by their intercourse with the sick, or exposure to the same atmosphere. The power to do this should exist somewhere, if it does not already; and, as the City Councils have no wish to increase their own, they could not but approve, were the Board of Health to acquire it for themselves and successors, under such regulations as would forbid the abuse of it. The suppression of the threatened epidemic of last Summer, "in more than one position previously to the accession of frost," if not attributable to some atmospherical vicissitude, may be ascribed to the decisive measures adopted by the Board of Health; and the fact so encouraging may induce the Legislature to strengthen their hands, in anticipation of a similar emergency. But while that Board is disposed to add to their duties those following the increase of power, your Committee feel assured that Councils will be no less vigilant on their part to enact such ordinances as may come in aid of those of the State.

The cleanliness of a city ought to be a primary object with its representatives, especially in our climate, since it is agreed on all hands that a pure atmosphere is no less desirable as a mean of preventing the spread of malignant fevers, than as a certain alleviation of them. Various schemes for improvement in our ordinances connected with this subject, may be developed occasionally; but your Committee cannot forbear to urge a few of the most important, for immediate consideration, and with a view to the reference of some to Select Committees. Those schemes are founded on such facts as have been communicated, or are known, and your Committee recommend—

First. That alterations in the present mode of contracting for cleaning the streets and alleys, be adopted; it appearing to your Committee, that while the contractor is entitled to the street dirt as part of his emolument, he will gather it from the places most convenient for himself, before he sends the carts to the narrow courts and alleys, though, for the promotion of general health, the earliest attention should be given to these. And your Committee would invite the attention of Councils to an ordinance of New York, prescribing the terms of their contract for cleaning. The ordinance divides that city into two districts; provides for contracting with one or more persons in each district, for collecting and carrying away *all* the filth at *stated periods;* obliges housekeepers to place the offal of their houses in the street on certain days and hours, *and at no others;* prohibits the keeping of such offal, or casting it into back yards and alleys; causes the contractors to remove filth from the market houses in certain days and hours; and forbids all persons, except contractors, from carrying away street dirt. There is another ordinance of New York, which appoints an inspector of hidden nuisances; this, with some additions to extend his duty to the discovery of nuisances in public streets, and to making report to the contractors, who may be subjected to penalties for neglecting to remove such nuisances upon notice given by the inspector, your Committee recommend as a precedent for one of our own.

Second. That *all* alleys leading into public streets be taken under the public superintendency, if authority from the State may be obtained—the right of the Corporation now extending only to such alleys as are twenty feet wide and upwards; that narrower alleys be paved by the owners, and in default thereof, that they be closed at their intersection with the streets, or paved by the public, the expenses to be assessed on lots adjoining the alleys.

Third. That some mode may be adopted for using the hydrant water *at the same time* when the scavengers are at work; and that hydrants, for this purpose, be placed on the highest situations in the city plot.

Fourth. That in future, hewn stone shall be laid for a bottom, as well as a side of gutters, in order to give a clear passage for water and filth, and to prevent damage done by brushing or picking with the broom, the gravel or sand from between the pebbles or bricks with which the gutters are now paved, in consequence of which, large holes are made—the receptacles of filth.

Fifth. That no wharf shall be hereafter built unless the dock on either side be so deep as to be covered by water at low tide.

Sixth. That docks now made, and which are not covered at low tide, be filled up or dug deeper to produce that effect at the head of the dock.

Seventh. That wharves be paved by the owners, and cleansed as the streets are or shall be, and that, when paved, they shall be raised above the summit of spring tides.

Eighth. That privies shall be sunk to gravel, or to the depth of—— feet, where there is none.

Ninth. That no tavern license be granted or removed, in any part of the city, unless the lot has sufficient space outside of the house for a privy.

Tenth. That no tavern licenses be hereafter granted for any houses, except those now licensed, and ferry houses, from the east side of Front street to Delaware river, inclusive. This recommendation is predicated on the fact, that our *summer pestilence* has generally commenced and raged with greatest violence within those limits; where the houses are built most closely to each other, where the streets are narrowest, where the greatest degree of dampness is uniformly present, where the tortuous direction of streets obstruct perflation, confining heat, moisture, and effluvia from filth in conjunction, and where, consequently, the exciting causes of fever, arising from intemperate drinking, would multiply victims to that disease. This limited prohibition of licenses would have the further desirable effect of preventing many stangers and others from being exposed, in certain seasons, to a morbific atmosphere, during the usual hours of repose.

Eleventh. That inquiry be made respecting the best means of regulating the number of inmates or boarders in one house, where that number is so great, in proportion to the space for accommodation, as to endanger its health or that of the public.

The annexed communications from Medical Societies, the Board of Health, and individuals, as well as the public testimony of a late Committee of citizens, prove the existence of nuisances unheard of before the present investigation, which obviously require the active interposition of the constituted authorities.

A plan for their suppression, and for other purposes, has been recently published by a gentleman, distinguished for his philanthropy and enterprise, commended by many, and urged upon the notice of councils by medical men of all parties. Deeply sensible as your committee are, of the beneficial and permanent effects on health to result from its completion, there are considerations attending it which restrain them from a full examination of its merits. Nor is the plan so well understood by all the advocates of its general tendency, as to present distinct parts for deliberation; and if it were, the corporation is not competent alone to accomplish it. The Legislature, the Judiciary, the patriotic supporters of the scheme, and the individuals to be affected by its adoption, the Board of Health, and the Wardens of the Port, should be consulted. Moreover, it is acknowledged to be capable of amendment; it will receive its perfection from the hands in (which) it rests. Time will be necessary to make it worthy of the unequivocal patronage of its friends, whose activity and zeal might be checked by any interposition of councils. But alterations are *now* required in the eastern section of the city, which councils should, in the opinion of your committee, attend to without delay—which pertain to their province, and are within their means; some of those may require the aid of a court of law, and of the Wardens, as, if a special committee should deem it expedient (and your committee deem it indispensable) that a new street, fronting the stores on the wharf, be laid out, and the wharves extended. To affect this, the court should be applied to for the power; the Wardens, for their opinion of its bearing on the river channel; and the councils, for the means of paving it. And if the improvement of that section be so important as your committee believe it, they cannot perceive a more suitable place for a beginning than the water side, for a new paved street there, raised high enough to prevent spring tides from extending to the cellars or the ground floors of buildings, would be a certain convenience, an additional mean of promoting health, and a help to more extensive schemes for meliorating the climate of that vicinity.

The labor of collecting necessary information previous to the designation of the street, the conference with individuals concerned, and applications to the court would, with other business to be presented in that particular district, occupy all the time that could be reasonably required of a committee, and your committee, therefore, recommend—

Twelfth. That a committee of three from each council be forthwith appointed, to inquire into the most expedient measures for improvement in that part of the city eastward of Front street, with a view to the preservation of the general health.

JOHN R. COATES,	JOHN M. SCOTT,
B. TAYLOR,	J. W. THOMPSON,
C. WATSON,	ELIJAH GRIFFITHS.

February 8th, 1821.

A.

To JOHN R. COATES, Chairman of the Joint Committee of the Select and Common Councils, "appointed to inquire into the facts connected with the appearance and prevalence of malignant or pestilential disease during the past summer," &c., &c.

The College of Physicians of Philadelphia have deliberately considered the following questions proposed by you on the 29th November last, and have directed the replies thereto to be communicated to you:—

First. Most of the members of the College had an opportunity of observing cases of malignant fever in Philadelphia, during the months of July, August, September and October last. The type was as malignant as we have ever known it; those persons who remained in the infected districts, after having been taken sick, seldom recovered; remedies did not appear to have the usual effects in their cases.

Second. The Board of Health, from their more correct knowledge of the facts, are best qualified to give satisfactory answers to these particulars.

Third. The disease, though malignant, was partial. It gave way on the appearance of frost, but not in that striking manner which had occurred in years when it was more widely spread.

Fourth. During the months of June, July, August, and September, every vessel from the coast of Africa, the West Indies, and the Continent of America, to the southward of Cape Fear, should undergo a strict search, and perform an effectual quarantine. This procedure should take place during the whole year with respect to vessels from the Mediterranean.

To prevent the spreading of malignant fever amongst us, the Board of Health should have full power to remove vessels, and persons, and to prevent communication with infected places; also, to have infected houses, bedding, and clothing, thoroughly cleansed.

And *lastly*, We would recommend a strict attention to the means of producing cleanliness, and a free ventilation, especially in those parts of the city near the Delaware, where the malignant fever has always made its first appearance. This cannot be done whilst Water street continues in its present confined situation, with the accumulated filth of many years, and for the most part without privies. We therefore strongly recommend the prosecution of the plan now in contemplation, of removing the whole of the buildings from the east side of Front street, inclusive, to the river, beginning at Vine and ending at South street, according to the original plan of William Penn, the wise and intelligent founder of our city.

By order of the College of Physicians of Philadelphia.

December 14, 1820. THOMAS PARKE, President.

B.

DEAR SIR:—Entertaining a conviction that the disease commonly called yellow fever may originate in foreign as well as domestic filth, the Academy of Medicine have instructed us to say, in reply to the communication which they have had the honor to receive through you, from a Committee of the City Councils, that in their opinion, the most effectual plan which, probably, at present could be executed, of preventing a recurrence of the evil, would consist in a more vigilant exclusion of foul vessels from hot climates, and in greater attention to cleanliness, particularly as regards the eastern front of the city.

It being understood hat the Board of Health will soon take up this subject, with a view to an application for some further legislative provisions, the Academy hold in reserve for a conference with that body, to which they have reason to believe they will be invited, the details of these suggestions.

Deeply impressed, however, with its importance, they cannot forbear to express to the Councils in the strongest terms, their approbation, as an ulterior measure, of the well-known proposal of Mr. Beck, under an entire persuasion, that it is pre-eminently calculated to afford security against the re-visitations of the pestilential forms of fever. To such conclusion they are led by the fact, that whether the yellow fever be of local origin, or imported, it has uniformly made its appearance on the water side of the city, where it is quite certain that a state of things only exists to generate or nourish it, and by proof scarcely less indisputable, that the disease has never prevailed to any extent west of Fourth street.

It remains for us only to add, that several of the members of the Academy had ample opportunities of seeing the disease last season; that it seemed to them to have assumed a character of unusual typhoid malignity, and that according to their observations, it did cease in more than one position, previously to the accession of frost. With the highest respect, we are,

Dear Sir, your most obedient servants,

SAMUEL JACKSON,
N. CHAPMAN,
ALEX. KNIGHT.

JOHN R. COATES, Esq., Chairman, &c.
Philadelphia, Dec. 23d, 1820.

C.

Philadelphia, Feb. 4, 1821.

SIR:—I observe in the daily papers, that a Committee of the Select and Common Councils, of which you are chairman, requst me to answer certain questions in reference to the malignant fever which prevailed in our city during the past summer and autumn. Compelled by the Health Law to reside at the Lazaretto, from the first day of June to the first of October in every year, I had not an opportunity, personally, of inquiring into the local causes which it is supposed gave origin to the fever. I do not think it necessary to communicate to you the information I have received since my arrival in the city, as it will be, or has, all been submitted to you by the Board of Health, and the respectable societies you have called upon, many of whose members have in person made all the necessary inquiries. Three cases of the malignant fever which occurred last summer, came under my notice. Two of them were of the first cases in the city, near Race street wharf; the third occurred in the Brig Martha. They were sent to the hospital at the Lazaretto, by the Board of Health.

I have but one object in writing this letter (in addition to the respect which I entertain for your Committee,) and that is, to call your attention particularly to the eastern front of the city. Its confined and filthy condition must be known to you. It appears to me that if some plan similar to that proposed by Paul Beck, Jr., could be carried into effect, the health of the city would be much improved. In the summers of 1819-20, the fever originated in that quarter. I will not attempt to determine on the practicability of the plan to alter the eastern front of the city. Time, at all events, will be necessary to its accomplishment. In the mean while, I strongly recommend the appointment of persons whose sole duty shall be to superintend the cleanliness of the eastern parts of the city. In the month of March or April they should commence, and personally inspect every store, warehouse, cellar, dwelling-house, and such other places where filth may generate; and have the power to remove all offensive or dangerous matter immediately. They should also, at least twice a month, during the summer and autumn, closely examine all suspicious places, and suffer nothing calculated to injure the health of the city, to remain within its limits. If such officers should be appointed, the Councils will, of course, in their wisdom, particularly designate their duties. Under such a system of management, and a corresponding attention to foul and sickly vessels at the Lazaretto, with the blessing of Providence, I sincerely believe that malignant fever might be banished from the city.

It was my intention to have submitted to you some observations respecting the operations of the Health Law at the Lazaretto, but I declined it on account of the Board of Health having presented a memorial to the Legislature to effect certain alterations and additions, which, if carried, no doubt will have an influence in protecting the city from malignant fever.

With sentiments of respect,
I remain your obedient servant,
GEO. F. LEHMAN,
Lazaretto Physician.

JOHN R. COATES, Esq., Chairman, &c.

D.

To the Joint Committee "appointed by the Select and Common Councils of Philadelphia, to examine into the facts connected with the appearance and prevalence of the malignant or pestilential disease during the past summer and autumn; and to report those means that they may deem best adapted to prevent its recurrence, or to check its progress."

GENTLEMEN:—Though I am convinced from the opportunities which I have had, at different times, of observing the rise and progress of the malignant or pestilential fever in Philadelphia, that it has been imported from the West Indies, I am also convinced that it is only propagated, or becomes epidemic in situations where the air is in a great measure confined, and rendered impure by the putrefaction of vegetables or other putrefiable substances; of course, the most certain method of preventiag its recurrence, is to subject all vessels arriving from the West Indies, and other places where the disease is prevalent during the summer and autumnal months, to Quarentine at the Lazaretto; and to prevent such as do arrive without due performance of Quarentine, from communicating the disease to the inhabitants of this city; the wharves should be improved; the docks kept perfectly free from putrefying substances of every description; and all the houses, stores, and materials removed from Water street, and the east side of Front street, if practicable, and if not, to have all the caverns and cellars filled up; Water street, as well as the docks, raised and firmly paved, and every substance liable to putrefaction, prevented from being landed or allowed to remain near the wharves or Water street.

To satisfy you that I am correct in my opinion, I take the liberty to refer you to the accompanying manuscript copy of the communication of the College of Physicians of this city to the legislature of this State, in the year 1806, at which time Drs. Kuhn and Wister were members of the College, and approved of it.

With sentiments of sincere respect and esteem,
I am, gentlemen, your well-wisher and fellow-citizen,
WM. CURRIE.

Philada., Dec. 6, 1820.

A copy of the communication of the College of Physicians of Philadelphia, to the State Legislature, in the year 1806.

"In the year 1793, the latter end of July and the beginning of August, a fever of a new and very alarming nature made its first appearance in Water street, between Mulberry and Sassafras streets; and all the cases of that fever were evidently traced for the first two or three weeks to that particular part of the city, or to persons who had intercourse with the sick in that neighborhood; after which, other parts of the city, the Northern Liberties, and the district of Southwark, became gradually affected with the same disease, and it was not until the arrival of hard frost that it subsided, after having proved mortal to nearly five thousand persons."

"About the latter end of July, in the year 1797, a fever of the same description again occured in this city. It was observed first in Penn, below Pine street, from whence, it progressed gradually to different parts of the city, and district of Southwark. It ceased on the arrival of hard frost, and occured again at the same season of the year, in 1798, 1799, 1802, and 1805, and every time in some part of Water strèet. The peculiarity of the symptoms, the remarkable inefficacy of the remedies which are usually successful in curing fevers which commonly occur in the same season of the year, in low, wet situations, rendered offensive by putrefying vegetables, with somewhat similar symptoms during the early stage, its great mortality and contagious nature, convinced us that it was a disease essentially different from any fever that ever had occured in this city from domestic causes, and we were convinced that the contagion by which it was produced, was imported into Philadelphia by some of the vessels which arrived at this port from the West Indies."

"The first appearance of the malignant or destructive fever, usually called the yellow fever, has never been observed among the marshy tracts to the south of Southwark, or to the south-west of this city, nor in the confined and filthy alleys, or brick-ponds, but always in the neighborhood of the wharves, or on the salubrious banks of the Delaware at Kensington, and near the places where vessels from the West Indies have arrived. In fact, it was traced every time that it occured in this city, since 1793, to the present year, 1806, to the vicinity of some vessel or vessels from the West Indies, or to persons or clothing connected with them."

"The principal peculiarities of the malignant yellow fever, are its con tagious nature, the rapid progress of its symptoms, and the mortality consequent on it; but in all our observations and practice, we have never known a case where the remittent or bilious fever of this climate have proved contagious, though we are aware that they are sometimes attended with violent and dangerous symptoms; but this striking characteristic of contagion being absent, they have never become an object of public dread or concern."

E.

To the Joint Committee of the Select and Common Councils, "appointed to examine into the facts connected with the appearance and prevalence of malignant or pestilential disease," &c., &c.

GENTLEMEN:—Although a member of the College of Physicians, who have already replied to your communication addressed to them on the 29th November last, I beg your permission briefly to state some opinions in reply to your fourth query, which have often impressed me as important; and allow me further to premise, that they are the result of considerable reading and observation upon the disease in question; having been much interested in the subject whilst a member of the Board of Health, during the years 1817–18–19. The query alluded to is, "What means should be adopted, with a view of preventing the recurrence, or of checking the progress of malignant autumnal fever in this city?"

Whether yellow fever is of domestic or of foreign origin, is yet an undecided question. Very able and distinguished medical authors still contend that it is an imported disease; whilst many, perhaps the majority of the profession in the United States, assert that it arises from causes existing among us. In the midst of this uncertainty, then, it is surely the safest plan to guard both supposed avenues to the disease; and the Health Law of our city is intended to answer these purposes; that is, to provide means for enforcing an effectual quarantine on all vessels from sickly ports, and preserving, as far as practicable, a pure atmosphere throughout our city, by obviating or removing those causes which load it with noxious effluvia.

To ensure the former, however, the Health Law requires improvement, which I have no doubt will be very judiciously pointed out by the present Board of Health, to whom one of your communications was addressed.

To ensure the latter, adequate power is not, nor cannot be, given to a Board of Health: other municipal authorities must come in to their aid.

I will proceed, then, to state three desiderata, which I have thought very important, as a means of preventing the recurrence, or of checking the progress of yellow fever in this city.

1st. To remove all the buildings included between Front street and the river Delaware.

Setting aside all disputes about the primary source of yellow fever, the history of the disease, I believe, in all situations where it has existed, has placed its first appearance on the wharves of seaport towns. And, with but very little well-attested evidence to the contrary, the history of the disease also goes to prove that it is *not communicable, or does not spread itself in a pure atmosphere.*

Whether, then, the disease be an imported one, and spreads from vessels on the wharves to the adjacent buildings through the medium of a vitiated air already produced, or arising from the holds of vessels, infected persons, clothing, or damaged cargoes; or, whether the disease be induced, in the first place, by the effluvia created by the accumulated filth and crowded condition of the buildings and their occupants on the wharves. In either case, would not the removal of these confined buildings, and the unavoidable filth produced by them, so long as they remain, ensure a free ventilation, and a pure air, and hence promise to be a very important preventive measure?

If the disease has a local origin in existing causes on the wharf, where it has always first appeared, surely the removal of those causes would give good grounds to believe that the alleged effects must cease.

On the other hand, if an imported disease, the removal of those causes which vitiate the atmosphere, prevent ventilation, and produce a medium fitted to convey it from the infected vessels at the wharves, would also give us a very reasonable assurance of an exemption from that source.—I sincerely hope, then, that the proposed plan of Mr. Beck, now so zealously advocated, will turn out a practicable one. I have long thought that if any *price* could make it so, it could scarcely be bought at too dear a rate. Before any proposition was before the public to effect this measure, I have repeatedly expressed an opinion that it would do more towards securing us from Yellow Fever than the present quarantine regulations.

2d. As a means of preserving a purer atmosphere throughout our city, I would propose the necessity of the Councils making it obligatory upon all owners of *privies* to sink them to water. The effluvia from ten or fifteen thousand privies, during the summer months, must add greatly to the impurity of the air we breathe in this city.

Any effect such an ordinance might have upon the water in the wells, would be of little consequence, as the Schuylkill water is now so universally substituted and preferred. Or, if a practicable plan, the objection to communicating the privies with the common sewers does not now obtain, that did formerly, or will not, at least, when the dam shall be completed across the Schuylkill at the Upper Ferry, as there will then be no water introduced which will have mixed with that of the Delaware.

3d. Another cause contaminating our atmosphere, and a subject of perpetual complaint in the summer months, is the filthy and offensive condition of our *sluggish gutters*. The Board of Health have no power over the Schuylkill water; nor if they had, is there water to spare for cleansing the gutters. But as we are promised a more abundant supply, when the plan now in operation for the purpose shall be completed, I would propose, as essentially important, that the Councils should provide for the erection of perpetual fountains, so situated as to insure the gutters constantly kept clean during the hot weather. These means, together with a strict attention to general cleanliness throughout this well built and well ventilated city, would, I humbly think, give us a warranted assurance that, with the blessing of the beneficial Ruler of events upon our endeavors, we should escape the awful disease which is the subject of your communication.

I am, very respectfully, yours, &c.,

SAMUEL EMLEN, JR.

January 1st, 1821.

F

To John R. Coates, Esq., Chairman of the Committee of the City Councils.

SIR:—The several queries you addressed to the Board of Health, on the part of the committee appointed by the city councils, were submitted to a committee, by whom the following answers to your respective questions were reported, and which we now have the honor to communicate to you:

1st. It being the special duty of the Board of Health to take cognizance of all cases of malignant fever in the city, it is scarcely necessary to say, in answer to your first question, that the Board has a knowledge of all the cases of that disease which occurred in this city in the months of July, August, September, and October, 1820.

2d. As it respects the general and local causes that existed in the parts of the city where the disease prevailed, and which may be conjectured to have had an agency in its production, we refer you to the accompanying paper, which is about to be published, in which all the facts in relation to that subject are detailed.

3d. The disease entirely disappeared at Hodge's dock and vicinity, before the occurrence of frost. The last decidedly characterized case in that locality was on the second of August. Subsequently to that period that portion of the city was as healthy and as free from diseases, as the city generally. The disease had also very considerably abated at Walnut street, before the appearance of frost.

4th. The fourth question, which regards "the means that should be adopted with a view of preventing the recurrence or of checking the progress of malignant autumnal fever in this city," is one of deep import and interest, and which, it is to be regretted, cannot be solved with absolute certainty. It is a subject which, for many years, has engaged the attention of our most enlightened and intelligent citizens, the most eminent members of the medical profession, and our legislative bodies; but no system that has yet been devised, has proved effectual in guarding our city from the disease, in periods that are propitious to its occurrence.

Our quarantine regulations and health system, are almost exclusively based upon the opinion, that the disease is always imported, and communicated by personal contagion and fomites, and that it cannot be generated from our own soil, and exists in our atmosphere.

While so great a contrariety of sentiment exists with those whose means and habits of observation, render them the most competent to settle this much controverted subject, it may well be considered as imprudent to trust to the accuracy of one only of the doctrines. To close up every avenue of danger, the possibility, that both may be true, should constitute the spirit, and govern the principles of the law.

In Gibralter this compound system of prevention has been adopted, and appears to have been completely successful. A most rigid internal police has been established, which has converted that port from being one remarkable for its foulness and filthiness, into one noted for its cleanliness and propriety—at the same time, a rigid exclusion from infected places, and a strict quarantine have been maintained. Under this two-fold and combined plan, Gibralter has been preserved from the ravages of malignant or yellow fever, although it has been repeatedly desolated with that disease, when protection was trusted solely to exclusion and quarantine, and while Cadiz, Xeres, and other neighboring cities of Spain, which rely solely on them for their safety, continue to be afflicted with that scourge. From these views, it appears to the Board of Health, that the best and most probable means to prevent the recurrence of malignant fever in our city, will be attained by amending the present health law, so as to render it more extensive in its principles, and more efficient in its provisions; at the same time a better arrangement of the police of the city, as it respects the maintainance of cleanliness, and the establishment of some regulations that will early abate existing nuisances, seems to be required of the corporation.

It is considered unnecessary to give a particular detail of the amendments deemed requisite in the present health law, councils having no jurisdiction in that particular. But we beg leave to direct your attention to certain duties incumbent on councils to perform, and powers which they can exercise, in doing which, they will essentially co-operate with and aid this Board in their exertions to preserve the health of the city.

1st. It is a common practice for the citizens to throw into the streets, in the summer season, the rinds of melons, parings of vegetables, husks of corn, and other vegetable and refuse matters. The scavengers seldom pass through any one street, more than once in two weeks, and consequently those matters accumulate in the streets, render them unsightly and filthy, become very offensive, and contaminate the air. This practice should be prohibited by ordinance, and carts be sent through the streets daily, at convenient hours, to collect and remove the various kitchen offals.

2d. The gutters, especially those in Water and Front streets, the alleys running from Water street to the wharves, and the steps communicating to Front street, should be washed and thoroughly cleansed, at least once a week in the warm months, with brooms, and by opening the fire plugs.

3d. Provision should be made for the early paving of the private streets, lanes, and alleys, of the city, and some plan adopted in order to compel the proprietors of property on them, to keep them clean.

4th. The deep docks that now indent the river border, and in which there is a constant accumulation of alluvion of the worst nature, should, if practicable, be altered, so as to have sluices, which might give a current through them; and the wharves, as soon as possible, should be paved, and faced with stone. To this end, it might be prohibited to construct any new wharves with logs, or to repair old ones with them. By this means, the present defective and very objectionable mode, in which our wharves are constructed, might, without being felt as burthensome by the owners, be gradually remedied.

5th. Privies and hog pens, especially the first, are a frequent and common cause of serious nuisances. At nearly every meeting of the Board, its attention is occupied with complaints preferred to them on this subject. In the warm months, the inconveniences arising from them are especially felt, and whole neighborhoods are infected by their noxious exhalations. Whether a very great advantage would not arise by the general introduction of the improved apparatus, proposed by a company in this city, and which has been adopted in Paris, London, and other large cities in Europe, may be worthy the particular consideration of your committee. Hog pens, if permitted in the city, ought to be cleansed at least once a day, in the warm weather.

6th. There is a species of nuisance of a disgusting character, productive of many evils, for which some remedy should be provided. Many houses in this city have no privies, nor any proper conveniences of that kind. On the east side of Front street, and in Water street, from Vine to Dock street, the Board have ascertained from examination, that there are about one hundred houses in which common open buckets are used, that are often emptied into the streets at night, or thrown into the docks. The landlords should be compelled to have some proper apparatus, when the rotary locality will not permit privies to be constructed, which will remedy a custom pregnant with so many evils.

It is believed that Councils have full powers to carry these necessary regulations into effect; but should it be thought otherwise, the Legislature would, doubtless, so enlarge the City charter, as to confer the authority to have them put in operation.

The plan for altering the eastern front of the city, as proposed by Mr. Beck, if it can be made practicable, appears to promise a reasonable expectation, that it would effect an exemption from this fatal scourge. It will be equally operative on either of the doctrines that are held, with respect to the disease. If it be of domestic origin, by removing and suppressing the numerous and unavoidable sources of vile nuisances, of confined and foul air, which must exist in that portion of the city as it now is, the disease must be effectually prevented from occurring. On the other hand, as it is very generally considered by those who believe the disease to be contagious, and to be produced by imported contagion, that it can only be propagated in confined places, and in an impure atmosphere, by procuring a free circulation of air, and establishing cleanliness, the disease cannot spread after it is imported.

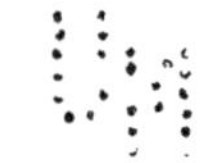

Besides, in the West India Islands, where yellow fever is unquestionably endemic, precisely the same as is noticed in this city, New York, Baltimore, &c., it invariably commences, and is generally confined to the water border, and does not first appear to prevail in those parts of the towns distant from the water. By removing the numerous inhabitants who now occupy the dwellings in that low, confined, and unwholesome situation, where the disease has invariable commenced its ravages, and which has always been its chosen and favorite seat, additional security will be gained against the origin or spreading of the disease when introduced. For it is the result of the most ample experience, founded on wide, extended, and accurate observations in various countries, that there is but little comparative danger of contracting a disease in an unwholesome or infected place in the day time. The great danger arises from being exposed to the cause of the disease in the damp air and dews of the night, and from sleeping in the poisoned atmosphere.

Whether the plan of Mr. Beck is practicable or not, is a question that is not considered necessary for us to examine. It is before the public, who are best able to determine the merits of the scheme, as well as the propriety of its execution.

When the disease has once made its appearance, the experience acquired in this city during the past summer and autumn, and in New York in the preceding year, furnishes the most ample and satisfactory proof, that the immediate removal of the inhabitants from the district infected, preventing access to it by the erection of barriers, and freeing it from all nuisances that might occasion noxious exhalations, are quite adequate to prevent its progress, and even to effect its total suppression.

With sentiments of respect,

Your obedient servant,

SAMUEL JACKSON,

Philada., Jan. 29, 1821. *President of the Board of Health.*

www.ingramcontent.com/pod-product-compliance
Lightning Source LLC
LaVergne TN
LVHW021414110826
845150LV00007B/1920

* 9 7 8 1 4 2 5 5 1 0 2 1 3 *